AFTER THE RAIN

Overcoming **DIABETES,
LUPUS,
ARTHRITIS,
SARCOIDOSIS,
PREDNISONE,
OBESITY**

AFTER THE RAIN

Overcoming **DIABETES,
LUPUS,
ARTHRITIS,
SARCOIDOSIS,
PREDNISONE,
OBESITY**

David Dobson

Library of Congress Control Number: 2009908662
ISBN: Hardcover   978-1-4415-6757-4
                 Softcover   978-1-4415-6756-7

This book was printed in the United States of America.

To order additional copies of this book, contact:
Xlibris Corporation
1-888-795-4274
www.Xlibris.com
Orders@Xlibris.com
64637

Contents

Introduction

The problem with getting sick is that everyone you know immediately becomes a physician. The more acute your illness becomes, the more specialized your friends become in your particular illness. To make things worse, the more that you ignore your friends prescribed cures, the more they insist that they know exactly how to cure your woes. Every sentence out of their mouths begins with, "What you need to do is . . . . ," and then prescribe, in detail, everything that will cure you.

Of course, every time that you do not blindly follow your friends expert opinion, they take it as a personal insult, not to mention, the more that you don't follow everyone's advice, the bigger the idiot that you are for not listening. When you are ill, it is difficult to listen to someone who has not experienced the same conditions that you are experiencing, even when it comes to your doctor. I am hoping that people with health conditions can identify with what I went through and will be encouraged to try to overcome their illnesses as opposed to simply just live with the illness. When I was 38, I was told that I would not see 40. I am 45 years old now and I feel better than ever. I feel so vibrant and young that I have to remind myself how old I am, I am still very young at heart.

I am not a doctor (I am an architect) and I will not tell you what you need to do, nor will I pretend to diagnose your health issues, I will simply tell you how I overcame very serious health problems and point you into the direction of what many people have discovered to help, if not cure their health issues.

As always, prior to starting any diet, lifestyle changes, exercise regimens, etc., consult with your healthcare physician.

The reason for writing this book is simple; there are so many complications with diabetes, lupus, sarcoidosis, and obesity that my doctors never warned me about. A lot of the information in this book comes from the answers to many questions that I have had over the years and have asked various medical experts in an effort to learn more about what was happening to my body. There are so many side effects of prednisone that my doctors never told me about. There is a simple cure for diabetes and autoimmune diseases that many people do not know about. I am hoping that people that are experiencing these complications will be helped by learning from my personal experiences, from one patient to another.

The reason for the title, "After the Rain," is simple. I used to live in San Diego, California, "America's Finest City," and always enjoyed watching the sunsets on the beach. The sky is always clearer and the sunsets more beautiful after the rain.

Chapter 1

The making of an eternal optimist, a brief autobiography

I have always been an optimistic person for as long as I can remember. I am neither a "glass half full" or "glass half empty" type of person, to me, the glass is always full. Even if it's just full of air, the glass is full of something. Sometimes I think I was just born that way, but for the most part, we are who we are because of our experiences in life.

People who know me say that I am always smiling, always happy, and a very pleasant person to be around. I am a child at heart, I try to keep a hold of that youthful idealism that we all had when we were kids. I also like to think of the motto of the unit I was in when I was in the Army, "Fortune and misfortune are the same to a man with a stout heart." That is the way I saw things when I was faced with the very serious health issues that I have endured over the past 8 years.

I really am glad for the way that I grew up. My father was in the Air Force throughout my childhood until my junior year in college. I was born at Robbins Air Force Base in Georgia. I was too young to remember living there of course, but I always remember a story my mother told me. My mom was going to our neighbor's house to borrow a cup of sugar when a stranger came by the house and asked for a drink of water. She let the man into the house and went to our neighbor's house. When she came back to the house, the man was gone, but she found that I had climbed on top of the stove, with my hands and knees on each of the burners and my twin sister had turned on all the burners. Thank God it was an electric stove.

I also have a sister that is three years older than me. According to my mom, my sister used to pick me up by my head when I was a baby. Maybe that explains why my neck is sore today.

When I was two, we moved to Vandenberg Air Force Base in Southern California. I got into as much trouble as any other kid, like stealing matches from the kitchen cabinets and setting a dumpster on fire and then have my mom throw me into the dumpster to put the fire out. I still remember my shoe laces catching fire.

At the age of 3, we got a dog; a mutt named Peanuts. My sisters, myself, and a lot of the neighborhood kids were playing in our front yard. My parents were outside watching us. Some kids came down the street with Peanuts in the basket of their bicycle, crying because they had to give her away or she would be taken to the dog pound. They asked us if we wanted the puppy, and my dad emphatically said, "No!" Of course, all of us kids pleaded with my dad, and he eventually caved in and we took in the dog.

When I was six, we moved to Karamusel Air Force Base in Karamusel, Turkey. Of course, by that time, Peanuts was a part of the family, and we took her with us. Right outside out back yard was an abandoned runway, and on the other side was a golf course and then the beach. We used to walk to the beach every day during the summer. There were no television stations there, so for all four years that we lived there, there was no TV. I can only imagine the trauma that going four years without television would cause children today. None of the kids in the neighborhood missed not having television, we always went out and played together.

When I was ten, we moved to Travis Air Force Base in California, just as cable TV was becoming commonplace. We were always active as kids, riding bikes, going to the pool, going to the playground, and of course playing with the neighborhood kids.

When I was twelve years old, we moved to Aviano Air Base in Italy, right at the foot of the Alps. This was an enjoyable time as we got to travel around Europe a lot. The base was rather small, and the high school contained grades 7-12 and only had around 200 students. During high school, I was so shy that if a girl came up and said hi to me, I couldn't say anything, I would just blush beet red. I had long hair at the time, as a lot of other people did in the mid 70's, and I have very curly hair. When I was a freshman, there was a girl that was a senior and she always called me "curly top." She would grab me in the hallway and kiss me on the forehead. I would be embarrassed and blush, while all the other guys in my class would be so envious of the red lipstick on my forehead.

At the age of fifteen, we moved to Barksdale Air Force Base in Bossier City, Louisiana. This was the first time that we went to a school off base, and it was the first time that I was exposed to racism. I could never understand racism and still don't to this day. I remember the first week of school there in biology class we learned about melanin, which is skin pigment. We all have melanin (except for albinos who have none), we just have different amounts of it. That is the only difference between everyone's skin color, so technically speaking, everyone has the same skin color.

I graduated high school in 1982 and went to college at the University of Texas at Arlington. The first day of college, they told us that even the best architects die broke, and that architects have a life expectancy of fifty-four because of the stress involved in the profession. So on my twenty-seventh birthday, I looked in the mirror and told myself that I made it half-way through and was glad that I still had all my hair. I still have it, only it's a bit thinner now.

Peanuts, our dog, died during my freshman year of college. I was very sad at first, but then I realized that she had had a great life, we had taken better care of her than I've seen some people take care of their children.

I came out of my shell in college and became very popular. Architecture school is incredibly demanding. The architecture building was the only building on campus that was open 24 hours, and there were always students in the building working on their projects.

I admit that I am not as talented when it comes to drawing as most architects are, and there is obviously a lot of drawing and design in architecture school. It seemed to take me twice as long to come up with a design that was half as good as everyone else in class. One of my professors told me in front of the class that I was the hardest working person in the class and that I may not have the natural talent that the other students had, but because of my work ethic, I would be a successful architect.

I also worked throughout my college days, which took time out of my afternoons and evenings for working on my school projects. Sunday, Tuesday, and Thursday nights were almost always all-nighters in order to get projects done for Monday, Wednesday, and Friday design classes. I would still be at my desk working when teachers and students would begin to arrive in the morning for classes. It was not uncommon to pull consecutive all-nighters during the week. The all-nighters that I spent focusing on my architectural projects took away from my other classes. I rarely had time to study for tests for my other classes and would be very happy to receive a "C." My second time through physics, I was happy to get a "D," at least it's a passing grade. My overall GPA was less than 2.5, but it was a very hard-earned less-than-2.5 GPA, I am not ashamed of it at all. Oh, the fond memories of those college days.

I graduated college in May 1987. I woke up one morning and it was time to graduate, the 5 years of college just blew right on by. Graduating from college was actually very anti-climactic, finishing the last final exam was where the real excitement was.

Like every college graduate, I sent resumes out by the dozens. My parents and sisters would help me scour newspaper want ads from all over the country. An architect from the Virgin Islands placed an ad in the Dallas Morning News, and without thinking, I sent my resume. The architect called me back and asked me to send a copy of my portfolio, which I did. A week later, he called me and offered me a job, which I eagerly accepted and told him I'd be there in two weeks. I immediately went into the other room and asked everyone if they knew where the Virgin Islands were because I had no clue and I had to be there in two weeks. I was very pleasantly surprised to find out I was moving to the Caribbean.

I moved to the Island of St. Thomas in the US Virgin Islands in September, 1987. It took me about 2 weeks to get acclimatized and had very little appetite, which was a good thing since, as a recent college graduate, I didn't have much money to eat with. My diet back in those days consisted of an apple and a carrot for lunch, and a baked potato and corn for dinner. When you are right out of college, you are more concerned about gaining experience than you are about making money. I either rode my bike or hitch-hiked to work. One day I rode my bike to work, and a very large cow that was walking on the side of the road suddenly decided to walk across the street. I hit the cow broadside, which felt like hitting a concrete wall. The cow ran off and I was left dazed on the pavement. If someone had had a video camera, they would have made a lot of money on America's Funniest Home Videos. But thankfully, for my pride's sake, nobody saw the collision.

The cow incident brought back vivid memories of the day I finally learned to ride my bicycle without training wheels when I was a kid. My parents, sisters, and I rode our bikes around the block with me in the front, I turned around to look back at everyone else, very proud to be in the front, then, wham!!! I hit a telephone pole with the side of my face. Just like the cow, I don't think the telephone pole felt the collision at all.

To go off on a tangent, I got hit in the face a lot in my life. All four years that I played Little League baseball, I got hit in the nose with the ball at least once per season. Maybe that explains why I am forty-five and have never been married.

In September 1989, Hurricane Hugo hit the Virgin Islands. It was a very long night as we experienced hurricane force winds for 12 hours as Hugo slowed down as it hit the Virgin Islands. I lost everything except for my car, which was parked right on the edge of a cliff.

A month before the hurricane, I had just moved into an apartment on the top of a 1500 foot mountain, with a view of the Caribbean Sea on one side, and a view of the Atlantic Ocean on the other. Incredible views on both sides. Right before the hurricane hit we closed the hurricane shutters thinking that it would be safe. I took inventory of all the food I had in my apartment and set out a bunch of canned food on my kitchen counter.

My best friend was the manager of a Christian radio station on St. Thomas, where I was also a part time DJ. I went to the radio station to ride out the storm, which may have saved my life. The hurricane was so powerful that it knocked the radio tower down and on top of the building we were in. Fortunately, the damage to the building was minimal and we were all fine. We were, however, trapped at the radio station for a few days as the fallen tower blocked the only road to the radio station.

We finally were able to get off the mountain that the radio station was on and made it to my apartment. A fifteen pound buoy had been carried by the wind from the harbor, and slammed through the hurricane shutters and kitchen window of my apartment and was sitting on the floor in the middle of the living/bedroom (it was an efficiency apartment). The broken glass had swirled around the inside of the apartment and was lying on the floor and on my bed. The screen from the kitchen window was embedded in the bathroom door. The swirling winds must have been very strong inside my apartment as the labels were blown off of the cans that I had left on the counter. The labels were still intact lying on the floor. But what was even more bizarre; I knew a couple that owned a Mexican restaurant on the waterfront. One of the tablecloths from their restaurant was carried up the 1500 foot mountain and was lying in my living room, next to the buoy.

Most of the houses in the Virgin Islands get their water from cisterns that catch rain water. Without electricity to run the pumps, houses do not have running water. We went weeks without power after the hurricane, and I know some people that didn't have electricity for two months after the hurricane. We all had to lower buckets down into the cisterns to get water to bathe ourselves, talk about having to take cold showers.

Since I was homeless after the hurricane, I stayed in an apartment at the radio station for a while, and then I moved into an apartment that had once been a laundry room. The ceiling was a half an inch shorter than me, I quickly learned not to stand up and stretch in the mornings.

The people of the Virgin Islands are very beautiful people. It was amazing to see everyone help each other rebuild after the hurricane damaged and destroyed much of the Islands.

When the recession hit the United States in the early 90's, it hit the Virgin Islands very hard as it is a tourist based economy. After months without a paycheck, my savings dried up and I had to do something immediately. I looked into the Army Corps of Engineers, but that didn't work out. I talked to the Army recruiter, who promised me that I would become an officer if I joined, so I decided to fulfill my childhood dream by becoming a paratrooper in the Army. Of course, I was not accepted into OCS as promised and I remained an enlisted man.

I went to basic training at Fort Leonard Wood in Missouri and then on to Airborne training at Fort Benning, Georgia. I received my jump wings on my thirtieth birthday, that was pretty cool, it made me feel like a kid again. I was stationed at Fort Bragg, North Carolina for all four years that I was in the Army.

My four years in the Army passed by very fast. My unit went to Haiti for a couple of months in 1994 as part of Operation Uphold Democracy. My unit built Camp Eagle, a base camp for the UN soldiers. Shortly after we left Haiti, a hurricane destroyed the base camp.

I took a part time job delivering pizza my last 2 years in the Army. I actually earned more money delivering pizza than what the Army paid me, which is pretty sad to say the least.

One night, while delivering pizza, it started raining as I drove down a winding two-lane road. My car started to fishtail as I approached a bend in the road. I quickly turned into the tailspin and my car turned in the other direction. Before I knew it, my car went out of control and I covered my face and head with my hands and held my elbows in together as they taught us to do in Airborne school. The window in the driver's door shattered and it felt as thought something was hitting the roof of the car. The car finally came to a stop and I just sat there in a daze. I looked outside my window and saw that I had come to a rest in a field in a field with tall grass. I looked to my right, and the spare tire, which had been screwed down in the back trunk, was next to my head over the passenger seat, as though it had been fixed to the roof of the car. I then realized that my car was upside down. I had gone off the road and rolled down a hill without realizing it.

Fortunately, I was able to climb out of my car and climb up to the road and was able to stop a passing car. Again, fortunately, there was a fire station less than 100 yards from where I had the accident. The ambulance got there within a few minutes and took me to the hospital at Ft. Bragg. Luckily, I had about a hundred small cuts and a lot of bruises everywhere, but nothing was broken.

I got out of the Army on my birthday in 1997; talk about an awesome birthday present. I stayed in North Carolina for 6 months after getting out of the Army and moved to Mission Viejo in Orange County, California on January 2, 1998 to continue my career in architecture.

Chapter 2

Living with Sarcoidosis

I was 35 when I moved to California. It seemed to me that it was time to buy a house and settle down. In May of 1998, I changed jobs and moved to San Diego, where I live today.

After living in San Diego for about a year, I woke up one morning and noticed a lump on the right side of my neck. It did not hurt at all, but I still made an appointment with my doctor immediately.

My doctor told me that the lump on my neck was more than likely a swollen salivary gland and if I sucked on some lemons, the gland would open up and the swelling would go down. She told me that it was nothing to worry about.

In June of 1999 I became ill and went to see my doctor again. The lump on my neck still had not gone down. My doctor diagnosed me with having a sinus infection and assured me that the lump on my neck was not associated with the sinus infection. She prescribed antibiotics for 10 days and the sinus infection went away within a week.

About a month later, I became ill again and went to see my doctor again. This time I was diagnosed with the flu and was again assured that the flu had nothing to do with the lump on my neck, which still had not gone down. After a week of antibiotics, the flu went away; however, the lump on my neck remained.

I then went to see another doctor about the lump in my neck. These doctors also told me that it was not anything serious and recommended some medication that I cannot recall now. Within another month, I became ill once again. The new doctor diagnosed me as having a sinus infection. He too prescribed antibiotics, and within a week, the sinus infection went away.

For the rest of the year, I became ill at least once a month. I was diagnosed with either the flu or a sinus infection, and each time I saw a doctor, they assured me that the illness had nothing to do with the lump in my neck. Around October, I began coughing a lot several times a day. This continued on through December. There was several times where I would cough uncontrollably and lose consciousness for a few seconds.

I went to Texas to spend Christmas with my parents, sisters, and their families. We all gathered for dinner on Christmas Eve at a restaurant, when suddenly my nose started running profusely. It would not stop running, no matter what I did to try to stop it, it just kept running like a faucet. When I woke up on Christmas morning, I felt so horrible that I went back to sleep after being up for only fifteen minutes. I later went to see a local doctor, and he diagnosed me with the flu and prescribed more antibiotics. For the rest of the week that I was in Texas, I was very ill and stayed in bed for most of the time.

By the time I got back to California after the Christmas break, I was constantly coughing, and at least once an hour I would cough up phlem and throw up due to the fact that I have a very bad gag reflex. By the end of the second week of January, I was throwing up three or four times an hour. I would start wheezing, which gave me about a two to three minute warning before I would cough up the phlem, and I knew that I had to get to the bathroom because I knew I would soon begin laughing at the carpet (the technical term for vomiting). This had an effect on my co-workers, as they could hear me throw up in the bathroom due to the echo caused by the tile on the walls. A lot of my co-workers complained to my boss about it and a few of them demanded that I get fired.

At the same time, a second lump appeared under my right jaw, and a third lump appeared on the left side of my neck. I went to two different doctors and a hospital emergency room those first two weeks back in San Diego. They all diagnosed me with the flu and prescribed antibiotics. The flu never cleared up.

I went to two more hospital emergency rooms, and both times I was told that they were too busy with flu patients and I should go home and take aspirin. From the middle of January to the middle of February, I went to eleven different doctors and hospital emergency rooms. They all told me that I had the flu and either told me to go because they were too busy with flu patients, or they would prescribe the same antibiotics that were not working.

I went to the VA hospital emergency room after work on a Friday as a last resort. I originally did not want to go there as I had heard that the VA had a bad reputation for being difficult to deal with. Immediately upon checking in with the nurse and telling her my story, she asked me if any of the other doctors or hospitals had an X-ray taken of my chest. I said, "no," and she told me to go directly to Radiology and they would be waiting for me. I walked down the hall to Radiology, thinking that it would take at least an hour to be seen. As soon as I walked in the door, the radiologist escorted me into a room and took X-rays of my chest. He told me to go back to the urgent care waiting room and the nurse would call me in immediately to see a doctor. Again, I thought, "Yeah, right, an hour or two will be more like it." As soon as I got back to the urgent care waiting room (a two-minute walk down the hallway), the head nurse was waiting for me and escorted me into an examination room, told me to take off my clothes and the doctor would be in to see me in a couple of minutes.

I had barely taken my clothes off, except for my undies (thank goodness I was wearing them that day) and four doctors and the nurse walked in looking at my X-ray and talking amongst themselves. They seemed perplexed and concerned by what they were looking at. They were all pointing to different parts of my chest X-ray and saying things like, "This is very strange," and, "This shouldn't be here," and, "This just doesn't look good."

Well, those who know me know that I am very light hearted and joke around a lot. I saw where one of the doctors was pointing on my X-ray, and I pointed to the same place on my chest, and asked, "You mean right here?" He looked at me and said, "Yes."

I said, "I've felt something strange right here ever since that night I was driving through the desert, I saw a bright light, and I woke up naked on the side of the road the next morning." All four of the doctors looked at me and cracked a smile, knowing I was joking around. The nurse, however, looked at me and asked, "What happened?" If only I could have taken a picture of her face; she thought I was serious and her mouth dropped wide open. It was nice to see the doctors smile as they had such serious looks on their faces.

They explained to me that all of the lymph nodes in my chest were swollen and they had never seen anything like it. They checked under my armpits and groin area and my lymph nodes were swollen there also. They had some blood drawn and told me that I would be called in for an examination early the next week. Before I left the hospital however, one of the doctors sat down and told me that the primary cause of my symptoms was AIDS. Since I do not use intravenous or any other type of drugs, nor am I homosexual, I was confident that I did not have AIDS and told the doctor that. He again told me that AIDS is the primary cause of my symptoms and I should be prepared for the worse.

Early on, when the doctors were trying to come up with a diagnosis, I was told that I had a low white blood cell count or I would be told that my red blood cells were denser than they should be. Every time I asked one of the doctors what that meant, they would beat around the bush and not answer my question.

For the next month, I had at least two or three appointments a week with different physicians at the VA in nearly every clinic. I had so much blood drawn out of me that it seemed that they were using me to single-handedly fill up the San Diego blood bank. I felt like a human pin cushion as they tested me for at least a dozen diseases. Every time I had an appointment with one of the doctors, they would always pull up a chair in front of me, look me in the eye and say, "Mr. Dobson, this is very serious . . . ," and proceed to explain to me that they could not determine what was wrong with me, and until they got the results of my AIDS test, they were preparing for the worse and thought that I should too. I would always try to lighten up the situation and I always told the doctors not to be so gloomy. One of the doctors at the VA told me that the heads of every department had a meeting every Monday to discuss unusual cases. He told me that I was the number one topic of discussion at those meetings since I had so much going on in my body.

One of the things they wanted to do was to perform a biopsy of one of my lymph nodes to see if it was cancerous. I also had small lumps that the doctors called granulomas on my chest that began to appear and the doctors wanted to perform a biopsy on one of the lumps on my chest.

A few days after the biopsy was performed, I had a follow-up appointment with my doctor. He told me that he and the other doctors were sure that what I had was a disease called sarcoid, and on top of it, I had a lung infection. My first thought was, "Leave it up to me to contract a disease that sounds like a damned video game." He told me that sarcoidosis is an autoimmune disease that is a multi-system disease, where the body attacks itself. The only way for them to truly identify the sarcoidosis was by ruling out all other diseases that can cause the same symptoms. My doctor told me that there was very little known of the disease, and the best way to treat it was by taking a steroid called prednisone.

As soon as I got home, I logged onto the internet and searched for any information on sarcoidosis. After searching for over an hour, I could not find much information on sarcoidosis. It was very frustrating being diagnosed with a disease and not being able to have any information about it. I had asked my doctor at the VA for more information but he did not have much to share. He did say that the medical profession does not know what causes sarcoidosis, but there was suspicion that it may be triggered by an allergic reaction or there may be a relationship between rheumatoid arthritis and sarcoidosis. I wanted to know more as my mom has rheumatoid arthritis but there was nothing more that he could tell me.

My doctor told me that there were several serious side effects of taking the prednisone and I would have to sign a waiver in order to take the medicine. At the time, I was feeling so ill, I was willing to take anything that would make me feel better. The only side effects that he told me of were the weight gain, particularly in the abdominal area and chest, hump back, and a feeling of euphoria. I told myself that if I started to get a hump back, I would stop taking it immediately. Fortunately, the hump back is one of the side effects that I did not experience.

I took the prednisone before even leaving the hospital. By the time I went to bed that night, I could tell that the lumps in my neck were starting to go down, and I wasn't coughing as much as I had been. The next morning, I was excited to see that all three of the lumps on my neck had disappeared. I also had the euphoric feeling that my doctor had told me about, I was feeling unusually energetic. When I walked, I had the euphoric feeling that my feet were not touching the ground, and my mind felt so clear that I could concentrate on anything I was doing without being distracted by anything.

By lunch time, I was feeling hyperactive and had to go outside for a walk. There was a road leading to the office park where I worked that meandered down a hill for about a half mile or so to an intersection with another road at the bottom of the hill. During lunch, there were several people in the office that would walk down to the intersection and back. This particular day, I walked down to the intersection and back, but I still felt like I had a lot more energy, so I walked down to the bottom of the hill a second time.

By 3 pm, I began feeling hyperactive again and left the office early to go to the gym. After exercising on an elliptical trainer for an hour, I went home and made dinner. By 8 pm, I was feeling so energetic that I could not sit still, so I walked a mile and a half to the beach and back. As soon as I got back, I showered and went to bed around 10.

At 11:30 pm, I was suddenly awakened by the sound of someone shouting my name. The voice sounded like my mother's voice, and it sounded as if she were standing right over my bed. I looked around, and obviously, didn't see anything, as I lived in San Diego, and my parents live in Texas. I went back to sleep, and a half hour later, I was awaken by the sound of the cabinets in my kitchen slamming shut. I jumped out of bed and ran into the kitchen to find nothing unusual. I went back to bed, and around 12:30 am, I woke to what sounded like a party in my living room. I walked into my living room, and again found nothing unusual. I walked out on my patio and noticed that there were no lights on in any of my neighbors units, and no sound other than crickets.

I woke up at 1 am and could not get back to sleep. I felt hyperactive and went out for a walk. I got back in at 3am and still could not go back to sleep. I went to the gym and spent an hour on the exercise bike and stair machine. I went home, showered, and went to work by 5 am.

This went on for a week. I would get to work between 4 am and 5 am, and go outside to take a walk every two hours because I had so much energy. Every night, I could only sleep for three or four hours, and I was constantly waking up to very odd sounds; alarms, voices, whistles, dogs growling, doors slamming shut, etc. It's a good thing that I am such a laid-back person, each time I was awakened by an odd sound, I would just think to myself, "Well, I know I don't have anything that sounds like that," and I would just go back to sleep. After a week of only getting three or four hours of sleep a night, I was so exhausted that I slept for eight hours straight without hearing anything. The next night, however, it all started again, only three hours of sleep and a lot of strange noises.

After being on prednisone for two weeks, I had a follow-up appointment with my doctor. I told him about the weird noises at night but he did not say anything. He scheduled me for a sleep study clinic a few days later. When I got to the sleep study clinic, I was told to wait in a small room with about a dozen school desks in it. There were six other people in the room sitting in the desks. After about five minutes of waiting for the doctor to come into the room, a man sitting in the front row of desks turned around and asked, "Does anyone else here hear noises at night?" The rest of us in the room said, "Yes," almost simultaneously, and everyone had a look of relief on their faces; I know I felt very relieved to know that someone else was experiencing the same thing. It turned out that we all were taking prednisone, and we were all hearing weird noises at night.

To make a long story short, I participated in a sleep study test and was diagnosed with sleep apnea. Sleep apnea is an episode where a person either stops breathing or their breathing is greatly reduced for periods of 10 to 20 seconds or greater during sleep. I was given what's called a C-PAP machine, which has a tube and a mask that you wear at night that puts positive pressure in the lungs while you sleep. With the C-PAP machine, I was able to get about five hours of sleep. I would still be woken up by weird sounds, but not as often as before.

A couple of weeks later, I had another follow-up appointment with my doctor. I again asked him about the weird noises and he told me that he did not warn me about the auditory hallucinations caused by the prednisone because not everyone experiences hallucinations while taking prednisone and he did not want to suggest them. My doctor told me that more than likely the hallucinations were induced by the prednisone; however, he wanted to be sure so he set up a referral to a psychologist.

I got to the psychologists office not knowing what to expect. The psychologist was very young, and I couldn't resist the urge to joke around when she was asking me questions.

"Do you hear people always talking behind your back?"

"No."

"When you walk through a room, do you hear people mentioning your name?"

"No."

"When you watch TV, do you feel that the people on TV are talking directly at you?"

"No," at this point I was trying not to laugh as I could not help but find this line of questioning to be a little humorous, especially with the extraordinary serious look on her face. I asked, "Are you serious?"

She said, "Yes, I am very serious," and then she went on to explain to me that psychologists do not normally have a sense of humor.

After scolding me for not being serious enough, she asked me, "Do you feel that the FBI is listening in on your telephone conversations?"

I could not resist, I said, "Oh no, it's not the FBI, it's the NSA that listens to all my phone calls, they keep a record of everything I say." I should have earned an academy award for saying that with a straight face.

"How long have you felt that they have been listening to your phone conversations?" She had a very intense look on her face now.

"Oh, for about five or six years now." It was getting more and more difficult to keep a straight face now, but I pulled it off.

Anyway, I found out that she was right about one thing. It seemed that she did not have a sense of humor and this subjected me to another hour's worth of questioning. Finally, her last question, "Do you know why you are here?"

"Yes, I have been having very vivid dreams since I started taking prednisone because of the sarcoidosis." I was tired and ready to leave.

Then she said, "You know that you do not fit the demographics for sarcoidosis."

Okay, that was it, I couldn't resist, "Well, deep down inside of me there is an African-American woman trying to get out." Another academy award please for keeping a straight face while looking her in the eye as I said it.

This caught her off guard, and she asked, "How long have you felt that way?"

"Ever since I moved to the Virgin Islands in 1987," I said as if it were obvious.

That was worth having to sit through another hour's worth of questions.

Chapter 3

Life With Diabetes

I would have appointments with my doctor at the VA about every 4 weeks. I would always have blood drawn a week or so before my appointments so that my doctor would have the results by the time I had my appointment. My health had seemed to stabilize under the prednisone and my weight had finally stabilized at 364 pounds (I weighed about 210 before I started taking the prednisone). As a matter of reference, my height is 6'2".

I had a doctor's appointment in October 2001, and my doctor said that everything had remained constant over the previous few months. My doctor of course was concerned about my weight and kept telling me to lose weight. I was getting quite a bit of exercise, but my weight did not go down. The records at the VA are electronic and seem to have a graph for everything. The graph of my weight mimicked the graph that showed the dosage of prednisone I was on. The higher the dosage, the higher my weight; the lower the dosage, the lower my weight would be.

A strange thing happened in the month of November 2001. I was on a project site with my boss and one of my co-workers, when suddenly, I would have to go talk to mother-nature once an hour. (For those who are not aware, "talking to mother-nature" is the technical term for "urinating".) It seemed very odd to me. I made a mental note to talk to my doctor about it at my next appointment, which was scheduled for early January 2002, just over a month away. I flew to Texas to visit my family for Christmas in the middle of December. On top of having to talk to mother-nature every hour, I became very thirsty and dehydrated all of the time. As the days went on, by Christmas Eve I was having to go to the bathroom every 15 or 20 minutes, and immediately afterwards I would run to the refrigerator to get something to drink. After drinking all of the water in the refrigerator, I would drink sodas and juices because I was so dehydrated. Little did I know, I was just compounding the situation. I called the VA in San Diego and talked to my doctor. He told me to immediately go to the nearest emergency room to get looked at.

My dad drove me to the hospital and I saw the doctor at the emergency room. They drew some blood and told me to fill a cup. The doctor was not amused when I told him that I needed to fill a gallon jug; a small cup just wasn't going to do it. I waited in the waiting room for about a half hour when the doctor called me into his office. He told me that my blood sugar level was over 1300 and he was surprised that I had not lost consciousness. The doctor told me that normal blood sugar levels were between 70 and 100. He also told me that people generally pass out when blood sugar levels reach 900. The doctor then told me that they were going to admit me to the hospital immediately.

On Christmas Eve 2001, I was admitted to the hospital. I was thinking that it would only be for a few hours for observation, however, the doctor was thinking several days for my blood sugar level to stabilize. I was hospitalized in the intensive care ward so that the doctors could keep a close eye on me. It was interesting at first, being hooked up to all of the machines. I noticed that every time I moved or stood up all of the lines on the digital displays on the machines would move. I got bored playing with the machines after my first five minutes in the intensive care ward. They of course had me hooked up to an intravenous drip, along with insulin and liquid prednisone. I had more weird dreams on the prednisone drip than I had had with the prednisone tablets I was taking. At least it was something different to keep my mind occupied while I was confined to my little room. I also learned that no matter how many games of solitaire you play on a laptop in a day, the computer wins about 95% of the time.

I was in the hospital for 4 days. After 3 days, they moved me out of the intensive care ward to a regular room. This time, I had a roommate. Only 15 minutes after the nurses moved me into the room, the other guy asked for his own private room. During those 4 days, I must have proposed to 30 nurses. They all turned me down with the same excuse, "I can't, it's against the rules." You would think that other patients had proposed to them judging by the quickness of their responses.

My fourth day in the hospital and the doctor finally came to my room to talk to me. This is the first doctor that I've seen since I was in the emergency room several days prior. The only thing the doctor said to me was, "You are as dry as a bone, you are a diabetic and you need to take insulin," then he left. A few minutes later, one of the nurses came in to talk to me. After once again refusing my marriage proposal, she gave me some syringes and a few bottles of insulin and told me that I needed to take 150 units of insulin a day, and then she told me I could leave. She did not give me instructions as to how to give myself the injections, I had to chase down another nurse in the hallway. This time I was told that I had to get a blood-sugar monitor and give myself injections twice a day.

I flew back to San Diego a few days later and went to see my doctor a few days after that. He sat me down and explained that diabetes was having an elevated blood sugar level, and one of the side effects of the prednisone is diabetes. He explained that that is why he was having my blood drawn so frequently was to monitor my blood sugar levels. He showed me the graphs on his computer screen. Between August and October 2001, my blood sugar had jumped from 104 to 700. Apparently the people in the lab did not notice that my blood sugar had spiked. He gave me instructions on taking the insulin and he also gave me a booklet to keep track of what I ate and my blood sugar levels. I was giving myself 150 units of insulin a day; 80 units in the morning and 70 units at night. My blood sugar readings in the morning were consistently over 500 and at night, it was over 700. My doctor quickly raised my insulin dosage from 150 units a day to 170 units a day and my blood sugar was still around 500 in the mornings and over 700 in the evenings. At this point, I was still taking 60mg of prednisone to treat the sarcoidosis.

By the spring of 2002 I would have to get up out of bed once an hour or so to go to the bathroom, and I would awaken in the middle of the night with muscle cramps in my legs and I would be extremely thirsty. I began drinking a lot of water before going to bed, and I would still wake up around 1 or 2 in the morning with extreme muscle cramps. The calf muscles would cramp up first, and while trying to work those cramps out, the muscles in the shins would cramp up, causing the leg to draw up towards my chest. The only way to work out the cramp in the calf is to point the toes, but pointing the toes aggravates the muscle cramp in the shin area. To work out the cramp in the shin area, you have to point your toes, which in turn aggravates the muscle cramp in the calf. This became a very painful and miserable nightly occurrence as it would take up to twenty or thirty minutes to work the cramps out. In the meantime I was drinking nearly a gallon of water a night and was still very dehydrated.

Around this time I noticed that my feet were always cold, which is very odd for me as I am always very warm, even when everyone else in the room is freezing cold. I would wrap a couple of blankets around my feet when I went to bed at night and my feet would still be very very cold. I was happy when eventually the cold sensation went away and I thought my health must have been improving, until one day I climbed into the hot tub and I realized I could not tell how hot the water was until I was almost knee deep in the water. This gave me the golly-wallies (the technical term for being scared).

During one of my doctor's appointments at the VA, my doctor told me that my blood sugar level was running up around 1100. She lowered my dosage of prednisone from 60mg a day to 20mg a day in an effort to control the diabetes. Within a week, my blood sugar had dropped to around 200 in the mornings and below 500 in the evenings, which was very good news indeed. I stopped waking up with muscle cramps and I did not have to get up nearly as often at night to talk to mother nature, and best of all, I stopped having weird dreams. Unfortunately, my cough started to come back and my lung function tests got worse as the reduction in the prednisone dose caused the sarcoidosis to flare up. As a result, after being on the lower dose of prednisone for nearly 3 months, my doctor raised my dosage back up to 60mg per day. It was not long before the frequent trips to the bathroom, vivid dreams, and muscle cramps dominated every night once again for me.

I also noticed that my vision was gradually growing blurry. One morning, around 3 am, I had to drive up from San Diego to Fresno, California. As I was driving north through Ontario, California, my vision was so blurry that I could not see the reflectors on the lanes of the highway clearly. My vision had gotten so blurry that the lines on the highway would dance around as I drove. It was a good thing that I was familiar with the area and that I drove through the urban areas at night when there was little traffic on the road.

By late spring/early summer 2002, my doctor once again tried to lower the dosage of prednisone in an effort to control the diabetes. This time, not only did the sarcoidosis flare up, my doctor told me that I was showing signs of lupus. The notorious butterfly rash appeared on my face, lesions appeared on the back of my calves, my skin became very sensitive to the touch, I began to have frequent bloody noses, and I was constantly tired. On the lower doses of prednisone, my blood sugar was low enough to allow me to have a full night's sleep, however, I would wake up in the mornings completely exhausted as though I had run a marathon and there was a thousand pound weight on top of me. It would take all of my energy just to roll over, getting out of bed became an arduous chore.

As if that were not enough, suddenly both of my arms would go numb from the shoulder on down to my fingers. The odd thing was, when my arms went numb, only the index finger and thumb would go numb on my right hand, and on my left hand, only my pinkie, middle finger, and ring fingers would go numb. When my arms would go numb, I would not get the feeling back for up to 6 hours. The feeling would come back gradually from the shoulders down to the fingers. Little did I know at the time that this was the sarcoidosis affecting my nervous system. The doctors at the VA had subjected me to various tests to rule out carpel tunnel syndrome. I eventually noticed that if I lifted my head up, my arms would go numb within five seconds, however, that was not the only time I would experience the numbness, my arms would also go numb randomly with no noticeable cause.

With all of these symptoms, my doctor once again put me on 60mg of prednisone and recommended that I start taking methotrexate, another powerful drug. While the prednisone has immediate side effects, the methotrexate has more long term side effects. I had to sign a special consent form before taking the methotrexate. Once again, shortly after the increase in the dosage of the prednisone, the diabetes raged out of control, and I was back to the torturous nights of muscle cramps and frequent talks with mother nature.

I bought an exercise bike on an impulse one rainy day (one of the few days that it actually rained in San Diego) and set it up in my living room. One evening I took my blood sugar reading before riding the exercise bike. After an hour of riding the bike I took my blood sugar reading again and found that my blood sugar had dropped from 630 to 410. I started to take my blood sugar readings before and after exercising and found that my blood sugar level would drop around 200 points by the time I had finished exercising. I told this to my doctor and she told me that it was just a coincidence.

The first week of November 2002, a friend of mine in Florida e-mailed me a link to a seminar called, "Reversing Diabetes," that was going to be held in the Los Angeles area towards the end of November. I called the organization that was putting on the seminar and found out that there were going to be a lot of Seventh Day Adventist doctors at the seminars. I've known a lot of Adventists and I thought that if there was an alternative to prednisone, they would probably know about it. I immediately signed up for the seminar and became very eager for the day the seminar would start. I was like a child waiting for Christmas, I just could not wait for it. At the time, I didn't care at all about the diabetes; I was only thinking of finding an alternative for the prednisone. I knew that if the sarcoidosis didn't kill me, the prednisone would. At the age of 38 my doctor told me that unless something drastic happened, I would not see the age of 40.

Chapter 4

The Cure

The Reversing Diabetes seminar was scheduled to start on a Saturday evening at a resort hotel. I was so eager for the seminar to start, arrived about 4 hours before the registration even started. The seminar finally started and during the breaks, I would ask all of the doctors and nurses in attendance if they knew of an alternative to prednisone. Much to my chagrin, each one told me that there is no natural alternative. I was very disappointed but decided to stay at the seminar anyway. The seminar stressed a vegan diet and exercise. That sounded quite interesting, and they fed everyone very tasty vegan meals.

The next morning, on Sunday, I checked my blood sugar and was surprised when I saw that it was 216. It had not been below 300 since I was first diagnosed with diabetes. I thought I just took the reading wrong and ignored it. That day we sat in seminars, ate vegan meals for lunch and dinner, and took a walk after each meal.

The following morning, which was Monday morning, I tested my blood sugar level as always. I was totally shocked when my blood sugar reading was only 84; perfect. I couldn't believe it. I was totally excited. I tested it again to make sure I did not make any mistakes, and once again it read "84." I tested it yet again, and again the reading was "84." I tested it again, just to make sure, and the reading this time was "85." I was just so excited that I could not control myself. I ran down to the hallway outside of the conference rooms where some of the people running the seminar had gathered. I interrupted the conversation they were having and told them about my blood sugar level.

I was so excited that I told everyone in the seminar about it. Amazingly, as the first session of the day started, I noticed that I could see the projection screen a lot clearer, absolutely increadible.

The seminar lasted through late afternoon on that Monday. As I got into my truck and started driving away, I noticed something even greater: I could read the street signs and billboards. I hadn't really noticed how bad my vision had gotten until it had cleared up. It was now dark and I could see everything perfectly clear. It was like being able to see for the very first time. I drove slowly down the street reading all the street signs just because I could now see them. It was awesome.

I now thought that at least the diabetes can be kept in balance, but I still needed to find a natural alternative to the prednisone before the prednisone killed me. I had bought a cookbook at the seminar and went to the grocery store before driving home. The next morning, I put all the ingredients for lentil stew into a crock pot so that it would be ready for me after work. I even made scalloped potatoes from the cookbook for my lunch and took it to work. The scalloped potatoes were very tasteless but I ate them anyway knowing it was good for me. When I got home I was eager to try the lentil stew. I opened the lid and the lentil stew looked more like oatmeal than stew. It didn't taste that good but I ate it also, knowing that it was good for me.

The next day, I thought I would try the crock-pot lentil stew again only with less water. When I got home that night, it had the consistency of Thanksgiving stuffing. Well, I ate it again knowing that it would be good for me.

For the next few weeks, I kept experimenting with the recipes. I had not considered myself a good cook and these experiments proved that I indeed was not a naturally gifted gourmet chef. Every night after dinner, I would walk to the beach and back; 3 miles total. I began to have low blood sugar episodes and gradually lowered my insulin intake on my own as I would occasionally experience hypoglycemia; too low blood sugar.

My knees and ankles hurt because of the arthritis, but I was determined to get exercise. In the mornings, my ankles and knees hurt when I would get out of bed. One morning I noticed that they did not hurt as bad as they usually did. The next morning, exactly 3 weeks after attending the Reversing Diabetes seminar, my ankles and knees no longer hurt, and best of all, my blood sugar level was normal <u>without taking insulin</u>. Needless to say, I was very excited about it.

My next doctor's visit, I had blood drawn before seeing the doctor as usual. My doctor asked me how much insulin I was taking, and I said, "none." She then asked me what my blood sugar readings are when I take them, I said, "between 80 and 100." She then asked me again how much insulin I was taking, and, with a big smile, I said, "none." She then said, "Well, let me look at your lab work, that won't lie to me." She looked at her computer screen, then looked at me and again asked me how much insulin I was taking. I told her once again that I had stopped taking insulin on my own. We would repeat this conversation for the next few months. My doctor could not believe that I no longer had to take insulin and my blood sugar was normal.

My doctor had still wanted me to take prednisone and methotrexate. Since my health felt much better, I started lowering the doses of prednisone and methotrexate on my own. By three months after going to the Reversing Diabetes seminar, I had stopped taking the prednisone and methotrexate and my lung function tests were still improving, the lumps in my neck never came back, and my cough never came back.

One of the great things about the VA is it's efficiency. Now days I can have my blood drawn at the lab on the ground floor, and by the time I get to my doctors office, she will already have the results on her computer. The VA also keeps track of patient's prescriptions and automatically mails out refills. The VA kept mailing me bottles of insulin and packages of syringes. I kept telling my doctor that I no longer needed the insulin but she didn't believe me. It wasn't long before I had over two dozen bottles full of insulin in my refrigerator and a cabinet full of syringes. It took almost four months for the VA to stop mailing me the insulin and syringes.

Weimar Institute, which had put on the Reversing Diabetes seminar has a 3-week program where they feed you a vegan diet, provide consultations with doctors, provide massages and classes regarding general health, specifically diabetes, in a very serene setting outside of Sacramento, California. I went through this 3-week program four months after going to the Reversing Diabetes seminar. I highly recommend it to everyone. By the time I finished the 3-week program, my blood pressure had dropped to 116/63; perfect. I had always been concerned with high blood pressure as it runs in my dad's side of the family and my blood pressure had always run a little high. Today, it is no longer a concern for me.

Words cannot describe how thankful I am for the Reversing Diabetes program and the Weimar Institute. Looking back at how bad my health was, even I find it hard to believe that all that ill health was cleared up so quickly by diet and exercise. There is no doubt in my mind that having a good positive attitude has a lot to do with it as well. I know several people that are extremely pessimistic and I cannot help but think that if they were faced with the same health problems, they would have succumbed to it all.

I felt better than I ever had in my entire life. Everyone I know also noticed a big difference in me. Many people told me that I looked 100% healthier than ever; people told me that I got my color back. Apparently I had lost all the color in my face and had been pale for years.

Chapter 5

I Know Better Than This

Pride really does come before the fall. With our busy lifestyles these days it is easy to give in to the convenience of fast foods. It all started for me one night as I left work late at night and convinced myself that driving through a fast food restaurant just once would not hurt. Then it happened again a few nights later, then a few more times the following week until I was eating junk food several times a week on a regular basis. It all came to a head when I was faced with a very stressful situation with my mortgage. I was one of millions of Americans that had one of those bad adjustable rate mortgages that turned adjustable just after property values plummeted. I could not re-finance my house and the mortgage rate jumped from 6 ¼% to 9%, about $1,000 more a month. In six more months it was scheduled to jump up again to 14%. I tried every way imaginable to try to refinance my house to a fixed rate mortgage, but none of the banks or lenders would do it. I always pride myself on being a calm person that does not get stressed out over anything, but this was more than I could bear. I was under so much stress that I grew sores inside my mouth, I noticed that my hair was falling out, I was bleeding rectally, and suddenly, the diabetes came back in full force. It is amazing the effects that stress has on one's body. One week my blood sugar was normal, the next week it was back to over 500. I finally came to the conclusion that the only way out of my mortgage predicament was to default on the loan, the absolutely last thing anyone wants to do. The night that I concluded that defaulting was my only solution, I felt at peace and was finally able to sleep well at night for the first time in weeks.

By the next day, the sores in my mouth went away, the bleeding stopped, my hair stopped falling out, but because I had strayed from the vegan diet, the diabetes did not go away once I had dealt with the stress.

This time the diabetes lingered for a few months. Because of my previous success, I had become lackadaisical when dealing with the diabetes. One day at work, I got up to go talk to mother nature when suddenly I could not walk straight. I had instantly developed a bad limp. I had very bad balance and had to hold onto the wall as I walked down the hall to the bathroom. That evening I realized that I could not run anymore. After taking only one running step I would struggle to keep my balance just to stay standing. My doctor had never before told me that diabetes can interfere with neurological impulses.

I had always gone to the gym regularly, but suddenly, after only a few minutes on the elliptical trainer, I would become very lightheaded. I used to be able to go for an hour on the elliptical trainer between levels 12 and 15, but suddenly I could not even go five minutes at level 2 without getting very lightheaded. I would have to sit down for a few minutes to regain composure.

I realized I had become way too proud and had to immediately get serious and get back to what I know works. My doctor explained to me that since I had a history of diabetes I would be prone to it and I will always have to be careful and watch what I eat.

One day I was giving one of my nieces a piggy-back ride, my niece announced to everyone within a 10-mile radius, in a very loud voice, "I see Uncle David's bald spot!" As a typical male, I am both concerned and living in denial about hair loss. I had noticed that my hair had been becoming very thin but chalked it up to getting old. Of course I explained to my young niece that nano-sized aliens were abducting my hair follicles and taking them back to their spaceship to transplant onto Elvis' head (follicle abduction; you heard it here first).

In actuality, after talking to my doctor, hair loss is another symptom of diabetes. This alone should cause men everywhere to take diabetes seriously.

The company I worked for sent me to work in Kabul, Afghanistan. It took several weeks to find out that we could get many kinds of fresh fruits and vegetables. In fact, the fruits there were always very fresh and very sweet.

As I began to get back into the vegan diet, the limp became less and less severe until I could hardly notice it myself.

When I first started cooking I had no idea what I was doing. Now I have become quite proficient at cooking and often receive compliments when I cook for others. I used to have to follow recipes item by item; now I am to the point where I can experiment and create my own recipes. Instead of poisoning myself with junk, I now prefer to feed myself natural foods that actually taste very good. When I eat all natural foods I can feel the difference and I can see the difference in my health.

Chapter 6

Know Your Body

Before we learn about the effects that diabetes and other diseases have on our bodies, it is important to understand how various organs and systems in the body work and the importance of each.

At one time in our lives, many of us have learned about anatomy and biology in school. We learned about our major organs and the immune system and their functions. If you are like me though, you forgot about them right after taking the tests in school.

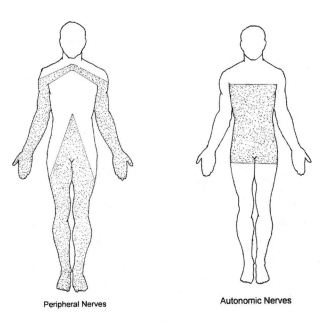

Peripheral Nerves   Autonomic Nerves

THE BRAIN / NERVOUS SYSTEM

The brain is the command center of the body. The brain weighs about 50 ounces in the adult male and about 45 ounces in the adult female. The brain is the command center of the body. The brain weighs about 50 ounces in the adult male and about 45 ounces in the adult female. From the brain, signals and impulses are carried throughout your body by the central nervous system that causes muscles to act and react. The brain also causes the secretions of chemicals and hormones throughout the body.

The human body has one single and highly integrated nervous system. For convenience we divide the nervous system to two parts. The first one is the Central Nervous System (CNS) which consists of brain and spinal cord. It is the integrating and commanding center of the nervous system which means CNS interprets incoming sensory information and dictates and organizes responses to the received sensory information. The second component of the nervous system is the Peripheral Nervous System (PNS). Everything outside of the CNS is a part of the Peripheral Nervous System. It consists of the nerves that extend from the brain and the spinal cord. The PNS has two functions. The first one is the sensory function which carries the impulses both from inside and outside the body to the Central Nervous System. And the second is the motor function that carries the impulses from the Central Nervous System to other parts of the body. The Nervous System is the controlling and communicating system of the body. It is responsible for all behavior performed by our bodies. It receives the information from the outside world and from within our body, interprets the signal and finally generates and executes the appropriate output.

The nervous system is broken down into four sets of nerves, the cranial, central, peripheral, and autonomic nerves.

The Cranial nerves run from the brain to the rest of the head. The central nerves run throughout the brain and spinal cord, the peripheral nerves run from spinal cord, to arms, legs, hands, and feet and the autonomic nerves run from spinal cord to lungs, heart, stomach, intestines, bladder, penis, and vagina.

Dysfunction of the nervous system can be impairing to the quality of one's life and contribute to severe illnesses.

THE HEART / CIRCULATORY SYSTEM

The heart is a muscle about the size of an adult fist, is located in the chest cavity. The heart is the pump of the circulatory system and has four chambers in it: the left and right ventricle and the left and right atrium. Blood carrying oxygen from the lungs enters the heart via the pulmonary arteries and is then pumped through the aorta artery and then through smaller arteries throughout the body. From the arteries blood flows through capillaries into the tissues of the body where oxygen and nutrients are absorbed into the body's tissues. Blood comes into contact with all cells within the body. Blood then flows from the capillaries into the veins and then flow back to the heart. This blood that now carries carbon dioxide passes into the right atrium and the right ventricle and then to the lungs via the pulmonary arteries.

THE LUNGS/PULMONARY SYSTEM

The lungs sandwich the heart in the chest cavity and supply the body with oxygen. The lungs are quite elastic and contain on average between 57 and 282 cubic inches of air in the average adult male during inhalation and exhilation.[1] As we breathe, on average of about 20 times per minute, give or take, oxygen is diffused from the lungs to the pulmonary capillary and oxygenates the blood. Oxygen is then carried throughout the body in the blood stream. Refer to the cardiovascular system for more information.

THE STOMACH

The stomach primarily stores the swallowed food and mixes it with acid that it produces to break down the food for digestion. The inside of the stomach walls are lined with mucosa to protect the stomach from being dissolved by the digestion process. The hydrochloric acid that the stomach creates not only aids in the digestion of foods, it also protects the body by killing viruses, bacteria, and parasites. The stomach then slowly pushes the food into the small intestine for further digestion. It takes between 4 to 5 hours for the stomach to totally empty its contents into the intestines. It is therefore recommended

---

[1]   Leonard, C. H., AMA, MD. The Concise Gray's Anatomy. 1997. p 180.

to allow at least 4 hours between meals. I have been told by my doctor and by several nutritionists that when new food is deposited into the stomach while the stomach still contains remnants of a previous meal, the stomach will begin to break down the new food until it reaches the digestive stage of the previous meal before the previous meal continues to be digested.

THE LIVER

The liver is about 10-12 inches by 6-7 inches by about 3 inches thick and weighs 3-4 pounds. The liver creates a brownish-yellowish fluid called bile, which is excreted through ducts into the small intestine for the breaking down of food and absorbing and digesting fats. This bile is stored in the gallbladder until it is ready to be pumped into the small intestines. The liver also stores nutrients and filters and processes chemicals in food. The liver plays a critical role by regulating blood glucose levels and supplying it to the other organs in the body. The liver also plays a critical role in the metabolism of carbohydrates. Glucose is used as fuel by the liver and is transported to the liver from the intestinal tract via the portal vein.

THE PANCREAS

The pancreas lies horizontally inside the abdomen behind the stomach. It is 6-8 inches long by 1 ½ inches in breadth by ½ inch thick. Pancreas produces insulin and glucagon which regulate the glucose (sugar) in the blood. The pancreas also creates enzymes that help the digestion process by breaking down proteins, carbohydrates and fats. The pancreas stores on average 200 units of insulin and secretes between 25-30 units of insulin per day in the average person.

THE KIDNEYS

The kidneys filter the blood through a network of blood vessels called glomuruli. This network of glomeruli form nephrons, there are about one million nephrons in each kidney. The kidneys filter out wastes substances, including urea while allowing water and nutrients to continue to flow through the circulatory system. Urea is later passed out of the body as urine. The normal amount of urine excreted by the normal adult is about 3 pints (about 1.5 liters).

The kidneys also regulate the volume of the blood as it circulates throughout the body. The volume of the body expands when large quantities of liquids are consumed resulting in more frequent urination as the kidneys attempt to keep the volume of the blood at steady levels. On the contrary, when not enough liquids are consumed, the volume of the blood is lower than normal and therefore the frequency of urination is lower.

Urine flows from the kidneys to the bladder via the ureters. Urine then flows from the bladder and is excreted via the urethra.

THE INTESTINES

Once food enters the small intestine from the stomach, glands from the walls of the small intestine secrete enzymes to break down the food even further. Additional digestive juices and enzymes from the pancreas and liver are also introduced in the small intestine for the process of digestion. The inside walls of the small intestine have folds in them that are covered with villi and microvilli that capture carbohydrates, folic acid, protein, sodium, calcium, vitamins, etc. More importantly, the intestines absorb the nutrients from food and they absorb water. The folds in the small intestine slow down the passage of food to increase the absorption of the nutrients.

The small intestine is about 20 feet long while the large intestine is about 5 feet long. The large intestine terminates at the rectum which is about 6 inches in length.

THE IMMUNE SYSTEM

The immune system is a minutely complex series of specialized cells and organs within the human body that protects the body from infections and diseases by recognizing foreign substances (antigens) and kills them or removes them from the body. White blood cells in the bloodstream destroy harmful substances such as viruses and bacteria that attack the body. The white blood cells perform several functions, one being the production of antibodies that respond to specific antigens. An autoimmune disorder occurs when the antibodies mistake the body's own natural healthy tissue for a foreign invader and attacks it.

The lymphatic system is an intricate part of the immune system and is intimately connected to the circulatory system. The lymphatic system is a series of ducts that carry fluid called lymph. Along the lymph vessels are enlarged masses of tissue called lymph nodes that contain tissue and are packed with lymphocytes (white blood cells) and phagocytes (cells that engulf and attack invading organisms. Lymph nodes act as filters that entrap particles and remove them from the bloodstream. When infection or disease occurs within the body, the lymph nodes will swell up as the phagocytes try to fight off whatever is attacking the body. When the lymph nodes swell up, doctors may conduct a biopsy of the lymph nodes to check for cancer as the lymph nodes would swell up as the phagocytes attack the cancerous tissue.

GLUCOSE

Enzymes in the kidneys, liver, small intestine, and platelets in the blood produces glucose during digestion. There are membrane insulin receptors on the exterior walls of the cells in body that act as doors for glucose to enter the cell. Insulin allows the glucose to be absorbed by the cells in the body. Once the glucose enters the cell, glycolysis oxidizes the cell to form energy for the cell.[2]

What Happens When We Eat

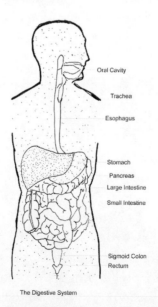

Oral Cavity

Trachea

Esophagus

Stomach
Pancreas
Large Intestine
Small Intestine

Sigmoid Colon
Rectum

The Digestive System

2   Levinthal, Gavin N., M.D., and Tavill, Anthony S., M.D., FRCP, FACP. <u>Liver Disease and Diabetes Mellitus</u>. 1999. Clinical Diabetes, p73, Vol. 17 No. 2

Before we even bite into food, our nose smells the aroma of the food, which sends signals to the brain, which in turn sends signals to the salivary glands in the mouth, which begin to secret saliva in the mouth. Once we bite into the food, the salivary glands secret even more saliva, mixing it with the food that makes the food easy to swallow. Our teeth bite and grind the food as the tongue mixes it with saliva, which contains enzymes that begin to digest the food. As we swallow the food, the food slides into the esophagus and is pushed down by a series of muscle contractions in the esophagus into the stomach. The pharynx guides the food into the esophagus and prevents food from entering into the voice box.

The stomach releases mucous, enzymes and hydrochloric acid that mixes with the food and begins to break it down in preparation for it to enter into the small intestine for digestion. The food is broken down and mixed with the stomach acids and enzymes to form a thick creamy substance called chyme. When the chyme is well mixed, muscle contractions send the chyme into the small intestine. The liver and pancreas secrete enzymes and juices into the small intestine through ducts that breaks down the food we eat into smaller molecules as it passes through the small intestine. The pancreas also produces insulin and glucagons, hormones that regulate the level of glucose in the bloodstream. The broken down food is then absorbed through the walls of the small intestine and into the bloodstream. The waste products of the digestion process are pushed through the large intestine and into the colon before being expelled from the body.

Chapter 7

Diabetes

Diabetes is the most prolific serial killer in the history of the planet. I remember as a child seeing television commercials raising the awareness of diabetes and the importance of funding research to find treatments for the disease. People without diabetes have no idea what it's like living with it. Many people that have diabetes downplay the disease and ignore its many symptoms and choose to simply live with diabetes day to day, which is very easy to do. It seems that Americans especially have the attitude that if we ignore something, it will go away. Diabetes will not simply go away. It continues to get worse and the condition compounds itself until the initial symptoms become severe.

There are two major types of diabetes; Type 1 and Type 2. Type 1 diabetes is commonly referred to as "juvenile diabetes," and Type 2 is the most common form of diabetes and is commonly referred to as "adult onset diabetes." There is a third type of diabetes called Gestational Diabetes, where during pregnancy, a woman's body is unable to produce an adequate amount of insulin.

Type 2 Diabetes is traditionally defined as a disease where the body's ability to produce or respond to insulin is impaired. Insulin is a hormone that assists blood glucose to enter the cells of the body. The blood glucose, also called blood sugar, is used by the cells as energy. Diabetes is characterized as an abnormally high level of glucose in the blood. There are many complications associated with diabetes as diabetes can affect many organs and systems within the body. Diabetes is a serious and deadly disease that affects millions of people and is an ever increasing epidemic. We are constantly bombarded with reports of the rampant spread of diabetes in the United States and throughout the world. The general consensus among the medical community is that there is no cure for diabetes.

People who are overweight are especially susceptible to diabetes. Fat in the body's cells make it difficult for the cells to allow glucose to be absorbed by the cells, increasing the amount of sugar in the blood, making the body's cells more resistant to insulin. I had a doctor that kept saying that diabetes has as much to do with fat as it does about blood sugar.

It is sad that many diabetics do not take the disease as serious as they should. I have talked to many diabetics that are very lackadaisical about diabetes. It seems that many diabetics are under the impression that as long as they take insulin they are fine. Some diabetics are convinced that as long as their blood sugar level is not too high, according to their own standards, they will be fine. Still others act as though if they ignore the problem, it will go away.

Sadder still, a recent news story indicated that many diabetics can no longer afford treatment and medication for their diabetes due to the recent economic downturn.[3] This will no doubt result in a sharp rise in diabetic complications and possibly lead to more deaths.

Yet, even sadder, there is a way to completely reverse diabetes without the use of drugs and expensive treatments, and most diabetics are not aware of this. It is simple, yet sometimes ignored when people are made aware of it.

Symptoms of Diabetes

TYPE 1 DIABETES

Frequent Urination
Excessive Thirst
Extreme Hunger
Sudden Weight Loss

---

[3]   Linda Johnson. *Diabetics skimp on lifesaving care in recession.* The Associated Press, April 12, 2009.

Weakness
Extreme Fatigue
Blurry Vision

TYPE 2 DIABETES

Frequent Urination
Excessive Thirst / Dry Mouth
Fatigue
Blurry Vision
Sudden Weight Loss
Erectile Dysfunction
Tingling or Numbness in Feet
Sharp Pain in Feet
Dry Skin
Vaginal Yeast Infections

The effects of diabetes on the body

LIVER

Diabetes increases the risk of liver disease such as nonalcoholic fatty liver disease (NAFLD).[4] Obesity is also closely linked to NAFLD.[5] In the majority of diabetes patients, there is a excess of glycogen accumulation in the liver. Type 2 diabetics are prone to an increase of fat stored in the cells of the liver in the form of triglyceride. This condition may progress to fibrosis or cirrhosis of the liver. Type 2 diabetics have an elevated risk of cirrhosis and liver cancer. A more advanced stage of NAFLD is called nonalcoholic steatohepatitis (NASH) where the inflamed liver cells can destroy the cells of the liver.

A survey conducted by the Department of Veterans Affairs and the National Institutes of Health show that the risk of liver disease and liver cancer in diabetics is double that of non diabetics.[6] A recent study has shown that there is a correlation between the risk of developing liver cancer and elevated fasting blood sugar levels.[7]

Diabetics have another concern to deal with. The introduction of insulin signals the liver to make cholesterol, which in turn adds to cardio-vascular disease.

HEART

High glucose levels in the blood leads to atherosclerosis, the build up of plaque on the inside walls of the arteries, veins, and capillaries. The buildup of plaque leads to resistance and constriction in blood circulation

[4] Collazo-Clavell, Maria, M.D. Diabetes: How does it affect my liver? 2008. MayoClinic.com. 6 October 2008

[5] Mendler, Michel, M.D. Fatty Liver: Nonalcoholic Fatty Liver Disease (NAFLD) and Nonalcoholic Steatohepatitis (NASH). 2008. MedicineNet.com. 10 October 2008 <http://medicinenet.com/fatty_liver/article.htm>

[6] Willocks, Jessica. Diabetes doubles risk of liver disease and liver cancer. 2004. Innovations-Report 13.02.2004.

[7] Preidt, Robert, Diabetes Boosts Liver Cancer Risk in Hepatitis, Cirrhosis Cases. June 5, 2008. MedicineNet.com. 10 October 2008 <http://www.medicinenet.com/script/main/art>

and also leads to the hardening of the arteries, where the arteries loose their elasticity. Hardening of the arteries contributes to high blood pressure and the clogging of small veins.

A heart attack occurs when a blood vessel leading to the heart becomes blocked. Not enough blood gets to the heart muscle and it becomes permanently damaged.

Atherosclerosis leads to high blood pressure, also called hypertension, which has been dubbed, "the silent killer," as it can eventually lead to heart attack and stroke. The increased resistance to blood circulation causes the heart to have to pump harder to pump the blood throughout the body. Diabetes doubles the risk of heart attack, heart disease, heart failure, and stroke. 65% of deaths related to diabetes are from heart disease.

Uncontrolled hypertension can lead to what is called end-organ damage, problems with the heart, kidneys, brain, eyes, and neurological damage. In some regions of the world, diabetics make up more than half of all patients with cardiovascular disease.[8]

Blood pressure is the measurement of the pressure of the blood in the veins when the heart pumps (systolic blood pressure) and again when the heart is at rest (diastolic blood pressure). Blood pressure readings are given as the systolic pressure over the diastolic pressure. Normal blood pressure is below 120/80. My doctor always told me that diabetics should keep their blood pressure well below 120/80. Everyone should check with their doctor regarding blood pressure and all health issues.

Stress and anxiety can cause a temporary increase in blood pressure. For example, my blood pressure now is normally around 116/63, but when I went to the dentist to get one of my teeth pulled, she measured it at 154/98. Back when I was a soda drinking carnivore my blood pressure was usually in the range of 130/90, dangerously high.

Renal hypertension is the constriction of the renal artery, the artery that supplies blood to the kidneys. As mentioned earlier, the narrowing of the renal artery is caused by the plaque buildup in the artery.

---

[8] Fontanarosa, Phil B., MD, MBA< DeAngelis, Catherine D., MD, MPH, Wong, John E. L., MBBS, FACP. JAMA, National University Health System, Singapore, Host Diabetes, Obesity Meeting. *JAMA The Journal of the American Medical Association.* October 15, 2008. 1750-1751.

Symptoms of hypertension include headache, dizziness, shortness of breath, and blurred vision. Other symptoms of heart disease includes chest pain and irregular heartbeat.

KIDNEYS

Due to the high amount of glucose in the blood stream, the kidneys become inflamed and do not filter the blood as they should. This is called diabetic nephropathy. This damage to the kidneys can lead to chronic renal failure, which will eventually require dialysis. Chronic renal failure can be slowed down if caught in the initial stages, however, it cannot be reversed. End stage renal failure is life threatening and may require kidney transplant.

FREQUENT URINATION

Urination is a normal bodily function with the purpose of removing toxins and waste from the body as well as excess water. Normal functions of the kidneys include the removal of urea from the blood as discussed earlier. When blood sugar levels get too high, the kidneys filter out some of the glucose with the urea and the glucose spills over into the urine leading to frequent urination.

Whenever my blood sugar level would get too high, I would have to urinate every hour, almost like clockwork. When it was extremely high, I would have to urinate even more frequently. Not only do diabetics have to urinate frequently, every time mother nature calls, they have to urinate more voluminously than normal. Not to be gross about it, but there have been numerous occasions where I would go for well over a minute, sometimes almost for two minutes (yes, I checked my watch out of morbid curiosity). There were times when I felt like I could read the entire newspaper while standing at the urinal.

Diabetes can lead to a bladder dysfunction called neurogenic bladder. This may cause the bladder to release urine unintentionally (urine leakage) or may cause the bladder to completely evacuate urine. This can lead to urinary tract infections.

One year I was traveling from Dallas to San Diego via Las Vegas on Superbowl Sunday. As the plane was nearing Las Vegas, I had a sudden strong urge to talk to mother nature. I wanted to wait until the plane landed, but there was another 15 minutes before we landed. I knew that I could not wait so I ventured to the bathroom, being tossed back and forth while walking up the aisle to the bathroom due to the amount of turbulence we were encountering. The flight attendants were very upset with me as we were about to land. The flight attendants wanted me to go back to my seat immediately, but I convinced them that since I had diabetes, I had to talk to mother nature right away or I would explode (probably not the best terminology to use on an airplane, but I needed to let them know that it was urgent).

The flight attendants, who were already strapped into their seats adjacent to the bathrooms, reluctantly let me use the rest room. In spite of the very bumpy ride due to the heavy turbulence, I did not miss my aim while I was bounced around the inside of the bathroom. When I was finished, I opened the door to the bathroom to go back to my seat, one of the flight attendants slammed the door shut on me and told me that I had to stay in the bathroom until we landed. I ended up closing the lid and sat down in the bathroom until we landed. I wish they had a seatbelt in the bathroom for me, it was a very bumpy ride.

DEHYDRATION

Diabetics also experience dehydration, mostly due to frequent urination. I would wake up at night with a very dry mouth and very dry skin. My mouth would be so dry that the skin inside my mouth would be stuck to my gums, and my tongue would be stuck to the roof of my mouth. Sometimes even my lips would be so dry that they would be stuck together. Only by drinking water and swirling it around inside my mouth could I get the skin and my tongue separated from the surrounding tissue. Even during the day I would be so thirsty when my glucose levels were high, that I would drink at least one bottle of water per hour to quench my thirst.

Keeping properly hydrated is essential for good health. Keeping hydrated will help the body flush out toxins and help keep the body functioning properly. As far as the digestive system goes, keeping properly hydrated soften the stools, which makes it easier for them to pass. On the contrary, it is difficult to pass stools while you are dehydrated, trust me on this, it is an unpleasant subject to talk about, and an even more unpleasant condition to experience.

EYES

Diabetic retinopathy, damage to the blood vessels in the eyes, results in blurry vision and can lead to blindness. Diabetes is one of the leading causes of preventable blindness.[9] Focal neuropathy, a type of neuropathy affects the cranial nerves that can lead to double vision or drooping eyelids. There can also be changes in how well your eyes react to light and dark.

Diabetes also increases the chances of developing cataracts and glaucoma.

LEGS AND FEET

Peripheral Arterial Disease (PAD) is the reduction in blood flow to the legs and feet caused by the buildup of fatty deposits. High glucose levels not only causes nerve damage (neuropathy), but can also cause cells in the legs and feet to die due to lack of oxygen and nutrients. Diabetics are prone to serious infections in the legs and feet and must take extra precaution in protecting them. Gangrene can set in, causing the toes, feet, and legs to be amputated.

The first step in treating this is to gain control of diabetes by bringing your blood sugar level down to a healthy level. The second step is to maintain a healthy blood sugar level through diet and exercise. Regular exercise can help relieve leg pain that many diabetics experience.

Diabetic amyotrophy is the deterioration of the thigh muscles. Diabetic amyotrophy affects the femoral nerve resulting in pain, weakness and eventual wasting away of the thigh muscles, beginning with the quadriceps. I lost a lot of muscle mass in the quadriceps, which obviously affected the amount of weight I could lift and my ability to jog and run.

Diabetics should take extra special care of their feet and inspect them every day, looking for cuts, blisters, sores, etc. Diabetics should wash their

---

[9]   Lerche, Jeanie Davis. 5 Steps to Managing Diabetes Complications. 2008. WebMD. 10 October 2008 <http://diatbetes.webmd.com/ diabetes-complications>

feet every day in warm water and dry them thoroughly, especially between the toes. When the feet are dry, diabetics should apply lotion or petroleum jelly on the feet.

Diabetics should always consult with their doctor regarding foot care and always protect their feet from injuries by wearing shoes, slippers, etc. Wearing socks or stockings will help protect against blisters.

Hydrotherapy is a good way to help encourage blood circulation in the feet and toes. First, soak your feet in hot water for about 3 minutes and then in ice cold water for about 30 seconds. The hot water should be as hot as you can stand it without causing damage to your skin. The hot water causes blood to rush to the feet and enlarges the blood vessels. The cold water causes the blood vessels to constrict and pushes the blood away from the toes. Repeat this 3 or 4 times, always end hydrotherapy with hot water.

Hydrotherapy is also effective in the shower in the same method. Set the shower water as hot as you can stand it, again without causing damage to your skin for 3 minutes and then turn the shower water cold for 30 seconds. This is good for general circulation and not specifically for increasing blood circulation in the feet. The previous paragraph is specifically for encouraging blood flow in the feet.

TEETH AND GUMS

Diabetes increases tooth decay and makes the body more susceptible to gum disease. I experienced a noticeable amount of tooth decay due to the diabetes. There are small gaps between my teeth that were not there several years ago. Infections in the gums can cause inflammation throughout the rest of the body.

THE BRAIN

One problem that can occur with type 2 diabetes is short term memory loss. My doctor and the doctors of many diabetes patients never mentioned this potential hazard of diabetes. I did notice that at times I would forget words or names that I should have known. I also noticed difficulty with my short term memory on occasions; typical signs of diabetes related cognitive impairments. I did not make the connection between memory loss and diabetes until I read it in a book some years after overcoming diabetes.

Premature memory loss occurs in diabetics due to the decrease in blood circulation caused by high glucose levels brought on by changes in cerebral insulin. When diabetics begin to notice memory loss problems, it is important to keep the mind stimulated through reading, crossword puzzles, etc.

HAIR LOSS

Follicle challengedness is probably the most distressing condition that men face. As the natural course of life goes, it seems that hair stops growing on the top of our head and it starts growing out of our noses and ears; ask any man in his forties. When the diabetes flared up after losing my house, I lost a lot of weight very rapidly and I noticed my hair becoming rapidly thin. Since the lupus and sarcoidosis were still in remission I just thought that the thinning of the hair was due to age. After a few months I realized that I was losing hair more rapid than my friends.

Diabetes and a poor diet both contribute to hair loss and premature balding. Daily hair loss is normal for everyone. Hair re-grows in the follicles on a regular basis. However, the loss or lack of protein and vitamins and minerals caused by diabetes can interfere with the reproduction of hair leading to the rapid thinning of hair.

NERVOUS SYSTEM (NEUROPATHY)

High blood sugar levels can damage all the nerves throughout the body over time. The longer that the blood glucose levels remain high, the higher the likelihood of developing neuropathy. 6 out of 10 diabetics suffer from neuropathy. The first signs of neuropathy usually occur in the toes, feet, and after a while, the lower legs. The constricted blood flow caused by diabetes to the nerves, particularly in the feet, legs, hands, and arms results in neuropathy. Diabetics often suffer from peripheral neuropathy, the sensation of cold, tingling and numbness in the extremities. Diabetics also experience sharp pain, as if being pricked by needles in the extremities due to neuropathy. Sixty percent of all diabetics will develop neuropathy.

Uncontrolled glucose levels can damage the covering on the nerves throughout the body and can also lead to more extreme forms of neuropathy such as interfering with the impulses from the brain throughout the nervous system. In my case, I developed a severe limp and suffered from impaired balance. I also lost the ability to stand on my toes and could no longer run or even jog. Right before developing diabetes, I used to be able to lift over 500 pounds (300 pounds plus my own weight) on the calf extension machine at the gym. After suffering from neuropathy, I could barely lift 50 pounds with my calf muscles. I have since recovered almost fully, I barely notice the limp and I can now almost lift as much as I used to be able to with my legs and I can now jog again.

Autonomic nerves may be affected resulting in dizziness, indigestion, belching, vomiting, diarrhea, stomach ache, and constipation. Heavy sweating and bladder control may also become problematic. Neuropathy can also result in Bell's palsy; the paralysis on one side of the face.

Damage to the autonomic nerves affects the beating of the heart and can cause blood to flow too slowly through the blood vessels. This damage also affects the digestive system, particularly the stomach and intestines. Damage to the autonomic nerves affect the sexual organs in men and women.

IMMUNE SYSTEM

Diabetics are especially prone to bacteria and infection. The immune system is constantly overwhelmed fighting the damage caused by high glucose levels. Diabetics are therefore more susceptible to colds, flu, and infections. High glucose levels also interfere with the involvement of the white blood cells in fighting antigens.[10] On top of this, diabetes suppresses the immune system, adding to the higher risk of diabetics developing infections.

---

[10] Kolatkar, Nikheel, M.D. Immune System & Diabetes. Your Total Health. 10 October 2008 <http://yourtotalhealth.ivillage.com/immune-system-diabetes.

STOMACH

Diabetes can lead to gastroparesis, a disorder where the stomach takes too long to empty its contents. The vagus nerves causes the stomach to contract and force food into the small intestine. As mentioned earlier, diabetes can damage the nervous system, and when the vagus nerve is damaged, food moves slower than normal through the digestion tract or stops altogether. This condition can cause the growth of bacteria due to the fermentation of the stagnant food. Gastroparesis is usually a chronic disorder but may be treated so that it can be somewhat controlled.

KETOACIDOSIS

Most commonly occurs in patients with Type 1 diabetes, but is also found in Type 2 diabetics. The body turns acidic as the body burns body fat uncontrollably and leads to ketone and glucose being passed in the urine when glucose levels get dangerously high. Symptoms of acidosis include nausea and chest pains. In my experience, it felt like an extreme case of acid indigestion, something that I had never experienced previously. Acidosis is often triggered by an infection. My experience with ketoacidosis occurred when I had an ear infection and led to being briefly hospitalized.

PANCREAS

Type 1 diabetes is a form of an autoimmune disease as the body's immune system attacks and kills the beta cells of the pancreas. The body does not produce additional beta cells, therefore, once all the beta cells are destroyed, the pancreas ceases to produce insulin. Symptoms of Type 1 diabetes will gradually manifest as the beta cells are destroyed and the pancreas loses it's ability to produce insulin. Occasionally, however, the symptoms of Type 1 diabetes will suddenly appear. Type 1 diabetics then need to administer insulin daily, which is why Type 1 diabetes is referred to as "insulin dependent diabetes."

Type 2 diabetes is referred to as insulin resistant diabetes. The body's response to the normal insulin produced by the pancreas is decreased, therefore, more insulin is needed. Insulin causes the body to store excess glucose as fat, which further inhibits the processing of previously stored fat. Injection of insulin therefore adds to the obesity of diabetics.

LIBIDO

In relation to the nervous system, diabetes can interfere with the autonomic nerves that control involuntary bodily functions, affecting the frequency and strength of erections (erectile dysfunction, also called impotence). Lack of blood flow caused by diabetes also has an effect on the ability to have and maintain an erection. Diabetics are more than 3 times more likely to suffer from erectile dysfunction. Other causes of erectile dysfunction include obesity, lack of exercise, lack of self esteem, drug use, smoking, and injuries and diseases. In addition to erectile dysfunction, diabetes can lead to retrograde ejaculation, where during ejaculation the semen goes into the bladder instead of out the penis. This condition is not harmful to the bladder as the semen is expelled along with the urine during urination.

Women may experience vaginal dryness or yeast infections due to diabetes. Autonomic neuropathy can also affect a woman's arousal, desire for sex, and feeling in the vaginal area.

Obesity also has an effect on libido. There is an inverse correlation between waist size and testosterone levels in men, the larger the waist size, the lower the levels of testosterone. Alcohol consumption and stress also lowers the level of testosterone in men.

SKIN

Diabetes causes dehydration through frequent urination. Dehydration can be tested by pinching the skin on the back of the hand and holding it for a few seconds and then releasing it. If the skin quickly returns to normal then there is probably no problem with dehydration. If it returns back to shape slowly then it is a sign of dehydration.

One affect that dehydration has on the skin is it can shrivel normally plump skin cells, creating lines and wrinkles prematurely. In my case, it seemed that wrinkles appeared overnight and new wrinkles and lines seemed to form every day. My skin also seemed scaly and itchy when my glucose levels were high.

Taking long, hot showers also contributes to wrinkles in the skin. To help prevent the signs of premature aging and wrinkles, it is important to keep hydrated, take less showers, and moisturize your skin.

COLON CANCER

According to Germany's Professional Association for Internists in Wiesbaden, individuals with Type 2 diabetes are 30% more susceptible to colon cancer. Diabetics are also more at risk of developing tumors. Diabetics are therefore encouraged to be screened for cancer.[11]

DIMENSIA

On April 15, 2009, USA Today reported on an article in the Journal of the American Medical Association that concluded that Type 2 diabetics face a great increased risk of developing dimensia.

With the exception of cancer and dimensia, I have experienced all of these diabetes related health challenges. It is my hope that diabetics everywhere will learn from my experiences and work to overcome diabetes.

---

[11] China Daily, In Brief, page 19. Cancer Check Must For Diabetics. September 10, 2008.

Chapter 8

Sarcoidosis

S arcoidosis, also called sarcoid, from the Greek words "sark" and "oid," meaning "flesh-like," is an inflammatory disease that occurs mostly in people between the ages of 20-40. Anyone can get sarcoidosis, however, the people that it affects the most are African American and Scandinavian women. It is also more prevalent in Asian, German, Irish, and Puerto Rican people than others.

The great comedian Bernie Mac passed away in 2008 at the young age of 50. Though the official cause of death was pneumonia, he had battled sarcoidosis for many years prior to his passing. This unfortunate event brought sarcoidosis into the limelight; the first time that many have heard of the rare disease.

Sarcoidosis is an autoimmune disease; it heightens the body's immune system, causing damage to the body's own healthy tissues. Sarcoid can appear in almost any organ and system within the human body; however, it most often affects the lymph nodes and lungs. The more common symptoms of sarcoidosis include chronic dry cough, skin rashes and/or lesions, including lupus pernio, weight loss, shortness of breath, fatigue, aches and pains, and inflammation of the eyes. Symptoms usually appear gradually as in my case; however, symptoms can also appear suddenly.

Sarcoidosis is a multi-system disorder. Symptons typically depend on which organ the disease affects.

General: About one third of patients will experience non-specific symptoms of fever, fatigue, weight loss, night sweats and an overall feeling of ill health. I didn't experience fatigue at first, but when the doctors lowered the dosage of prednisone and the sarcoidosis flared up, I experienced fatigue that is indescribable. After waking up from a full eight hours sleep, I would be so exhausted and weak that I could barely move, it felt like I had just ran a marathon and a giant weight was on top of me holding me down. It would take all of my energy just to roll over and crawl out of bed.

Lungs: The lungs are affected in more than 90% of patients with sarcoidosis. A cough that does not go away, shortness of breath, particularly with exertion and chest pain occur most frequently with the pulmonary form of the disease. At the time that I was diagnosed with sarcoidosis, I was also diagnosed with a lung infection. The cough that is caused by sarcoid is a dry cough. My cough was very productive due to the lung infection. About every fifteen to twenty minutes, I would cough up phlem, and with a very bad gag reflex, I would throw up.

Lymph nodes: Up to 90% of sarcoidosis patients have enlarged lymph nodes. Most often they are in the neck, but those under the chin, arm pits, and groin can be affected. The spleen, which is part of the lymphatic system, can also be affected. For over nine months, the lymph node on the right side of my neck was swollen and the doctors did now know what was causing it. The doctors kept telling me that the swollen lymph node was not related to the other illnesses I had at first. It was not until the VA X-rayed my chest and saw that all my lymph nodes in my neck, chest, and going were swollen that the doctors recognized the severity of my health.

Liver: Although between 50% to 80% of patients with sarcoidosis will have granulomas in their liver, most are without symptoms and do not require treatment.

Heart: Researchers estimate that cardiac sarcoidosis affects more than 10% of people with sarcoidosis in the US, and perhaps as many as 25%. Sarcoidosis can cause the heart to beat weakly, resulting in shortness of breath and swelling the legs. It can also cause irregular heartbeat.

Brain & nervous system: From 5% to 13% of sarcoid patients have neuralgic disease. Symptoms can include headaches, visual problems, weakness or numbness of an arm of leg and facial palsy. I had occasional numbness in both arms, but not at the same time. I would wake up with one of my arms completely numb from the shoulder down to the fingers. It was odd that the ring finger and pinky of my right arm did not go numb, and when my left arm went numb, everything but the middle and index fingers and thumb would go numb. My arms would go numb for several hours at a time and then the feeling would come back to normal. The doctors could not determine the cause of the numbness. The numbness has not come back since the sarcoidosis went away. I also had twitches in my face and at times thought I was having a stroke. I mentioned this to my doctors as well, and they could not explain why I was experiencing the twitches. Again, as soon as the sarcoidosis went away, I never experienced the twitches in my face again.

Skin: One in four of patients will have skin involvement. Painful or red, raised bumps on the legs or arms, called erythema nodosum, discoloration of the nose, cheeks, lips and ears, called lupus pernio, or small brownish and painless skin patches are symptoms of the cutaneous form of the disease. When the doctors reduced the prednisone to try to control the diabetes, a red rash formed on my cheeks and I got brown circular lesions on the back of my lower legs. The skin on my legs became very sensitive, if I brushed up against anything, it felt like the skin was being torn off, even if I just brushed up slightly against something.

Bones, joints & muscles: Joint pain occurs in about one-third of patients. Other symptoms include a mass in the muscle, muscle weakness and arthritis in the joints of the ankles, knees, elbows, wrists, hands and feet. When I got out of the Army, the VA told me that I would probably develop arthritis when I got older, so when I developed pain in my ankles, knees, back, and hands, I assumed it was arthritis, especially since my mom has rheumatoid arthritis.

Eyes: Any part of the eye can be affected by sarcoidosis and about 25% of patients have ocular involvement. Common symptoms include:

burning, itching, tearing, pain, red eye, sensitivity to light, dryness, seeing black spots (called "floaters") and blurred vision. Chronic uveitis can lead to glaucoma, cataracts, and blindness. I attributed my blurry vision to a changing prescription, however, my vision cleared right up in three days after going on a vegan diet. My vision had become very blurred for a while. My doctor told me that it was either because of the sarcoidosis or diabetes, but the black spots that I saw were definitely caused by the sarcoid.

Sinuses, nasal muscosa & larynx: About 5% of patients will have involvement in the sinuses with symptoms that can include sinusitis, hoarseness or shortness of breath.

Other organs: Rarely, the gastrointestinal tract, reproductive organs, salivary glands and the kidneys are affected by sarcoidosis.[12]

One particular characteristic of sarcoidosis is the formation of groups of microscopic inflamed cells called granuloma. Granuloma can form inside organs of sarcoidosis patients and can interfere with their normal function.[13]

The cause(s) of sarcoidosis are still not known. Researchers still have not determined what triggers the disease. Some people may have the disease and be asymptomatic. In other cases, it will effect people for a few years and go away completely on its own, while others will have occasional recurrences of sarcoidosis throughout the rest of their lives. Sarcoid can lead to blindness and occasionally may also become a severe chronic illness that can lead to death. There are only two other people that I know that have sarcoidosis. One of them is a white male and was diagnosed with sarcoidosis at the same age I was. He is now blind because of the disease.

The only other person I know that has been diagnosed with sarcoidosis was an African-American woman. Sarcoidosis had attacked her kidneys and her esophagus. She could no longer eat solid food and had to liquefy everything she ate. I have no idea how she is doing today.

---

12   Foundation For Sarcoidosis Research website
13   Foundation For Sarcoidosis Research website

When I was first diagnosed with sarcoidosis, it was widely believed to be hereditary in some way, which is why I was particularly interested when I heard that Karen Duffy of MTV was diagnosed with sarcoidosis as my mother's maiden name is Duffy. My doctors also told me that there may be a link between rheumatoid arthritis and sarcoidosis. My mom has been dealing with rheumatoid arthritis since I can remember.

Chapter 9

Lupus

Lupus is the most prevalent of many autoimmune diseases. Lupus is a chronic condition that can affect any part of the body. It is estimated that 1.5 million Americans have lupus and it affects women more often than it affects men. Like sarcoidosis, lupus is more prevalent in African-American women than Caucasian women, although all ethnic groups are susceptible to lupus.

Autoimmune diseases occur when the immune system cannot determine the difference between the body's healthy tissue and foreign invaders. The body then creates antibodies that attack and destroy the healthy tissues. There is no gene or group of genes that have been proven to bring about lupus. Like sarcoidosis, it is believed that genetics and environment plays a major factor in the development of lupus. Genetics make some people susceptible to the disease, which is triggered by something in the environment.

Although there are many lupus patients come from families with no history of lupus, many lupus patients come from families with a medical history of lupus or other autoimmune conditions. I was diagnosed with both sarcoidosis and lupus while my mother has rheumatoid arthritis and was recently diagnosed with lupus.

TYPES OF LUPUS

Systemic Lupus Erythematosus

Systemic lupus is the most common form of lupus. When people use the term "lupus," they often are referring to systemic lupus. There are several severe complications that can arise from lupus, including:

Lupus Nephritis, inflammation of the kidneys, which can hinder the kidneys' ability to filter waste from the blood. Lupus may damage the kidneys to the point that dialysis or kidney transplant may be required.

Pulmonary Hypertension, an increase of blood pressure in the lungs.

Inflammation of the brain and nervous system, increasing the risk of stroke and may cause headaches, memory loss, and confusion. Lupus may also cause inflammation of the blood vessels in the brain.

Coronary artery disease, the buildup of plaque on the inside of the artery walls.

Cutaneous Lupus Erythematosus

Cutaneous lupus erythematosus solely affects the skin and is associated with scaly red rashes. The most notorious being the butterfly rash across the nose and cheeks. Rashes associated with lupus come in the form of round, disc shaped rashes found mostly on skin exposed to the sun or fluorescent lighting, particularly on the scalp, face, and neck. Rashes can also develop on areas that are not generally exposed to the sun. I developed disc-shaped rashes, over 1/4-inch in diameter on the back of my lower legs (it was during the summer time when they first developed and I did work outside wearing shorts on occasion).

Drug-induced Lupus Erythematosus

As its name implies, drug-induced lupus erythematosus is caused by taking certain medications. The symptoms often mimic the symptoms of systemic lupus erythematosus, only this form of lupus normally does not affect any major organ. Normally, these symptoms will disappear within 6 months of cessation of the taking of the medication.

Neonatal Lupus

Neonatal lupus affects infants of women with lupus. This is a rare condition where the antibodies from the mother affect the child while in the womb. The child is sometimes born with skin rashes and liver problems, but usually recovers after a few months, while very few have a serious heart defect.

SYMPTOMS & COMPLICATIONS OF LUPUS

Since lupus can affect many different organs in the body, there are a wide range of symptoms. Lupus can flare up and go in remission at various times, therefore, symptoms may come and go from time to time.

Extreme fatigue: The fatigue associated with lupus is indescribable. I personally doubt that anyone without lupus can fully understand what this extreme fatigue is like. After getting a full night's sleep I still would be too exhausted to even move, getting out of bed was a major chore. I know several people suffering from lupus that would have to take naps just to remain functional during the day.

Cardiopulmonary system: Cardiovascular disease is a major complication of lupus; many lupus patients die of heart disease. Lupus causes inflammation of the pericardium, the sac that surrounds the heart. Symptoms include chest pain, particularly during deep inhalation. Lupus may also lead to anemia, a lower than normal red blood cell count and a low blood platelet count, resulting in bloody noses, easy bruising, and other bleeding disorders. Thrombosis is also a condition brought on by lupus, resulting in blood clots in the veins. Vasculitis, inflammation of blood vessels is also a condition brought on by lupus.

Brain and nervous system: Lupus patients have experienced problems with the central, peripheral, and autonomic nervous systems, due to inflammation of blood vessels, tissue, and nerves in an near the brain and nerves. Symptoms may be mild or severe and include headaches, confusion, tingling sensations, similar to carpel tunnel syndrome, fatigue, vision problems, seizures, facial pain, mood swings, depression, drooping eyelids, and gastrointestinal problems.

Joint and muscle pain: Lupus can cause pain and swelling in the joints like arthritis, the pain is usually the strongest in the morning but eases during the day. Lupus can also cause swelling in the hands, legs, feet, and around the eyes. Muscles my atrophy and lupus patients may have problems climbing stairs and ladders and may have trouble lifting objects and raising their arms.

Kidneys: Lupus nephritis is inflammation of the nephrons in the kidneys, which hinders the kidneys ability to filter waste out of the bloodstream. This in turn leads to waste buildup in the bloodstream, leading to swelling in the joints, hands, and ankles. Lupus nephritis can damage and scar the kidneys leading to end-stage renal disease, resulting in dialysis and transplants.

Skin rashes: Most notoriously, the butterfly rash on both cheeks. Other skin rashes occur in round-disc shapes (hence the term discoid lupus). These rashes are reddish and scaly, yet do not itch. The rashes that I experienced disappeared for good, without scaring, when the symptoms of lupus went into remission.

Eyes: Inflammation may lead to blurred vision, dry-eye, and uveitis, inflammation of the iris or other parts of the eye. Carticosteroids used to treat lupus and other autoimmune diseases may also lead to blurred vision and other complications with the eyes.

Hair loss: A little over half of lupus patients experience temporary hair loss that usually grows back with the treatment of lupus. Hair loss due to rashes on the scalp is usually permanent due to damage to the hair follicles. Hair loss due to corticosteroids used to treat lupus is also permanent.

TESTING FOR LUPUS

When lupus is suspected, doctors will order a series of tests to help with the diagnosis. An antinuclear antibody test (ANA) and anti-extractable nuclear antigen (anti-ENA) are the two main tests that are used. The ANA test detects certain antibodies in the bloodstream that are produced by the body's immune system. Lupus patients usually test positive for the presence of antinuclear antibodies, although lupus patients are not the only ones that test positive for antinuclear antibodies. Anti-Smith, anti-double stranded DNS, and anti-histone antibodies are the sub-antibodies that are specifically linked to systemic lupus

According to my doctors, physicians are reluctant to make a diagnosis of lupus. Doctors normally will not make a diagnosis of lupus unless at least 4 of the following 11 symptoms are present:

1 - Inflammation of the membrane around the heart (pericarditis) or inflammation of the membrane around the lungs (pleuritis).
2 - Ulcers in the mouth.
3 - Arthritis of the peripheral joints.
4 - Neurological disorders, including seizures, confusion, and psychosis.
5 - Renal disorder, protein or cellular casts present in urine.
6 - Hemotologic disorder, including anemia, thrombosis, among others.
7 - Positive ANA test, a blood test used to detect autoimmune disorders.
8 - Immunologic disorder.
9 - Butterfly rash (malar rash) on cheeks and nose.
10 - Discoid rash, scaly red non-itchy skin rashes.
11 - Sensitivity to ultraviolet light (photosensitivity).

Chapter 10

Arthritis

Arthritis is a broad term used to describe aches, pains, and inflammation, particularly in the joints. About 46 million Americans suffer from arthritis in one form or another. 60% of all arthritis sufferers are women. There are many types of arthritis; and each with its own cause. There are about a hundred different forms of arthritis, the two most common types of arthritis are osteoarthritis and rheumatoid arthritis. Over 20 million Americans suffer from osteoarthritis while between 1 and 2 million Americans suffer from Rheumatoid arthritis.

The joints, points where two bones come together, are naturally lubricated with cartilage, a mucous material that compresses when pressure is placed on the joint. The ends of the bones have tiny undulations in them, increasing the area of bone for the cartilage to bond to. The joints are lined with the synovial membrane, keeping the joints lubricated.

OSTEOARTHRITIS

Osteoarthritis, the most common form of arthritis, is also known as degenerative arthritis, degenerative joint disease, and wear and tear arthritis. Osteoarthritis however, is not solely due to wear and tear on the joints, it usually takes time to develop, which is why younger people generally do not suffer from osteoarthritis. Obesity and injury to the joints are also major contributors to osteoarthritis. The probability of developing painful osteoarthritis in the knee greatly increases with weight.

The primary symptom of osteoarthritis is sharp pain in the joints, sometimes described as a burning sensation in the tendons adjacent to the joints. Arthritis patients often describe a cracking noise, called "crepitus" when their affected joints are moved. When I was being bothered by arthritis, both of my knees made this cracking noise, especially when I would walk up and down stairs. It was loud enough for people to hear about 10 feet or more away from me.

Although any joint in the body can be affected, osteoarthritis usually affects the fingers, hands, knees, feet, toes, and spine, and hips. Joints in the fingers and toes may become enlarged. When my fingers became painful from arthritis, I would wrap my hands around an incandescent light bulb for the heat, which would help ease the pain for a while.

Osteoarthritis breaks down the cartilage in the joints. Cartilage is a slippery tissue that covers the bone at the joints and acts as a cushion between bones and absorbs the impact during movement. As the cartilage wears down, either by age, trauma, etc., the joints become painful. The hip and knee joints become especially painful upon walking and bearing weight. Losing weight can reduce arthritis pain in these joints. Over time, the cartilage between joints can lose resilience due to the dehydration of the cartilage itself. The causes of osteoarthritis include age, stress on the joints, obesity, wear and tear, injury, damage to or degeneration of the peripheral nervous system, loss of muscle mass, and even diabetes.

When I had my initial appointment with the Veterans Administration when I was getting out of the Army, the doctors told me that I should expect to have arthritis as I get older due to the wear and tear of jumping from planes. The military parachutes that we used are designed to bring down a 175 pound person at a rate of 17 feet per second. At the time, I weighed 205 pounds plus an additional 30-50 pounds of equipment that we carried. Needless to say, I, along with all paratroopers, had many hard landings. Fortunately, I never broke any bones or suffered any major injuries. The worst landing that I experienced was landing on one of my canteens on my tailbone, it hurt so badly that I couldn't sit down for a week.

RHEUMATOID ARTHRITIS

Rheumatoid arthritis is an autoimmune chronic inflammatory disease that primarily attacks the joints in the body, but can also affect many systems, tissues, and organs throughout the body, including the heart, muscles, skin, and blood vessels. Rheumatoid arthritis is a very painful, disabling, and frustrating disease. My mother has suffered from rheumatoid arthritis for as long as I can remember. When I first was diagnosed with sarcoidosis, my doctors discussed the probability of sarcoidosis being hereditary as sarcoidosis and rheumatoid arthritis are both autoimmune diseases.

In rheumatoid arthritis, the body's immune system reacts against the joint linings throughout the body. The synovium membrane around the joints becomes swollen and inflamed. This can also damage the cartilage between the joints. This often leads to constriction of movement of the joints and can cause the joints to be dislocated. Rheumatoid arthritis primarily affects fingers, wrists, knees and toes. The tendons and muscles can be damaged, leading to displacement of the joints. Many sufferers of rheumatoid arthritis, including my mother, have finger joints displaced sideways so that they do not line up with the forearm. Osteoarthritis affects the joints individually, rheumatoid arthritis affects the entire body.

(See "relief for arthritis sufferers" in Chapter 12).

Chapter 11

Prednisone

Prednisone is a corticosteroid, an immunosuppressant, meaning that it suppresses the entire immune system. As sarcoidosis is a disease that increases the body's immune system, prednisone is the most common treatment for sarcoidosis to suppress the overactive immune system. At first, I was so thankful for the Prednisone as all my symptoms diminished by the next morning, however, after taking the Prednisone over the following years, the side effects nearly killed me.

Some of the side effects of prednisone include the following:

Weight gain	Peptic ulcer
Facial swelling (moon face)	Infections
High blood pressure	Joint pain
Hallucinations	Cataracts
Diabetes	Insomnia
Mental confusion	Hyperactivity
Stretch Marks	Vivid dreams
Feeling of euphoria	Depression
Muscle twitching	Lightheadedness
Fatigue	Painful hips & shoulders
Osteoporosis	Abdominal pain
Blurred vision	Acne
Nervousness	Frequent urination
Increased appetite	Rash

Diarrhea   Cushing's syndrome
Kaposi's sarcoma   Seizures

The doctors at the VA had me come in once a month to draw blood and check up on me. The VA Hospital has their records on computer. My doctor showed me a graph that his computer generated, it showed the dosage of prednisone that I was on, my weight, blood pressure, and blood sugar level. My weight, blood pressure and blood sugar level followed the prednisone. When the dosage of prednisone went up, so did my weight, blood pressure and blood sugar level. When the dosage of prednisone went down, so did my weight, blood pressure and blood sugar level.

Weight gain by taking Prednisone is caused by the body retaining fluid due to the retention of sodium and losing potassium. Prednisone also causes an uncontrolled increase in appetite, contributing to weight gain. Once the prednisone dosage is lowered to below ten milligrams per day, the fluid retention and increased appetite will diminish, however, the weight that had been gained while taking the prednisone does not come off on its own. In a way it's fortunate that I am single, I can spend more time concentrating on getting a lot of exercise and I was able to drop the added weight rather quickly.

After taking prednisone for a week, the body becomes dependent on it and is no longer naturally able to synthesize natural corticosteroids. If a patient has been taking prednisone for a long period of time and suddenly stops, the body can experience an Addisonian crisis (a hormone deficiency caused by damage to the adrenal glands), which can lead to death.

Chapter 12

Obesity

"A high prevalence of overweight and obesity is of great public health concern because excess body fat leads to higher risk for premature death, type 2 diabetes, hypertension, dyslipidemia, cardiovascular disease, stroke, gall bladder disease, respiratory dysfunction, gout, osteoarthritis, and certain kinds of cancers."

U.S. Department of Health and Human Services and the U.S. Department of Agriculture, Dietary Guidelines for Americans, 2005

I will be the first to confess that while being obese, I lived in denial. Whenever I looked in the mirror I kept thinking that I really did not look that bad. I would often find myself comparing myself to others when I was out in public. It was not until I saw a photograph of myself that I realized just how obese I was.

Obesity is a rapidly growing epidemic, not just in the United States, but globally. According to a recent study, the percentage of people who are overweight or obese in the US in 2004 was 66.3%, up from 56.0% in 1991. During the same span, the number of overweight and obese in China climbed from 12.8% in 1991 to 29% in 2004.[14] I have had the good

---

[14] China Wrestles with Growing Obesity, USA Today, December 19, 2008, Page 16A.

fortune to travel to China several times over the last few years and have noticed that American fast food restaurants are becoming ever popular over there. I recently traveled to Singapore for work and noticed in the area that I stayed there was one McDonald's restaurant on every block, plus at least one other fast food restaurant. The recently published report, "F as in Fat," by the Trust for America's Health, states that two-thirds of Americans are overweight or obese.

> "During the past 30 years, adult obesity rates have doubled and childhood obesity rates have more than tripled."

> F as in Fat: How Obesity Policies are Failing in America, 2009.
> Trust for America's Health, Robert Wood Johnson Foundation,
> July 2009.

Being an Air Force brat I have had the privilege of traveling a lot while growing up. I love to travel and have been grateful for the opportunity to be able to travel a lot for work. It was always embarrassing to have to ask the stewardess for a seatbelt extension on the plane. To make things worse, being obese, my thigh would always push in on the button on the arm rest that reclines the seatback. During takeoffs and landings, I would have to wedge my hand between my thigh and the arm rest to keep my thigh from pushing in the button to keep my seat back from reclining back. Now, every time I fly, I am happy to see how much room I have with the seatbelt when I buckle up and have to tighten the seatbelt.

One of the worse things about being overweight is that almost everyone around you becomes a comedian. I heard all kinds of fat jokes imaginable. People I worked with would make comments and laugh hysterically. Making fat jokes is just not the way to encourage someone to lose weight, it only breeds resentment.

Obesity is the largest risk factor for Type 2 diabetes. Between 80 and 90 percent of diabetics are overweight. With the alarming rate in which our society is becoming obese, it is no wonder why diabetes is becoming the epidemic that it is.

Obesity can be simply defined as an excess of body fat. Body fat is measured by percentage. Generally, women with a body fat over 30% and men with a body fat over 25% are considered to be obese. In the United States, obesity has reached epidemic proportions with one in three Americans considered to be obese.

Another method to judge obesity is to use the body mass index (BMI). The body mass index equals a persons weight in kilograms divided by the persons height in meters squared (BMI = kg/m^2). A healthy BMI is generally between 19 and 25.

Body Mass Index

Categories: BMI 19–24 = Normal · BMI 25–29 = Overweight · BMI 30–39 = Obese · BMI 40–50 = Extremely Obese

Body Weight in Pounds — Height in Inches

Height (in) \ BMI	19	20	21	22	23	24	25	26	27	28	29	30	31	32	33	34	35	36	37	38	39	40	41	42	43	44	45	46	47	48	49	50
58	91	96	100	105	110	115	119	124	129	134	138	143	148	153	158	162	167	172	177	181	186	191	196	201	205	210	215	220	224	229	234	239
59	94	99	104	109	114	119	124	128	133	138	143	148	153	158	163	168	173	178	183	188	193	198	203	208	212	217	222	227	232	237	242	247
60	97	102	107	112	118	123	128	133	138	143	148	153	158	163	168	174	179	184	189	194	199	204	209	215	220	225	230	235	240	245	250	255
61	100	106	111	116	122	127	132	137	143	148	153	158	164	169	174	180	185	190	195	201	206	211	217	222	227	232	238	243	248	254	259	264
62	104	109	115	120	126	131	136	142	147	153	158	164	169	175	180	186	191	196	202	207	213	218	224	229	235	240	246	251	256	262	267	273
63	107	113	118	124	130	135	141	146	152	158	163	169	175	180	186	191	197	203	208	214	220	225	231	237	242	248	254	259	265	270	278	282
64	110	116	122	128	134	140	145	151	157	163	169	174	180	186	192	197	204	209	215	221	227	232	238	244	250	256	262	267	273	279	285	291
65	114	120	126	132	138	144	150	156	162	168	174	180	186	192	198	204	210	216	222	228	234	240	246	252	258	264	270	276	282	288	294	300
66	118	124	130	136	142	148	155	161	167	173	179	186	192	198	204	210	216	223	229	235	241	247	253	260	266	272	278	284	291	297	303	309
67	121	127	134	140	146	153	159	166	172	178	185	191	198	204	211	217	223	230	236	242	249	255	261	268	274	280	287	293	299	306	312	319
68	125	131	138	144	151	158	164	171	177	184	190	197	203	210	216	223	230	236	243	249	256	262	269	276	282	289	295	302	308	315	322	328
69	128	135	142	149	155	162	169	176	182	189	196	203	209	216	223	230	236	243	250	257	263	270	277	284	291	297	304	311	318	324	331	338
70	132	139	146	153	160	167	174	181	188	195	202	209	216	222	229	236	243	250	257	264	271	278	285	292	299	306	313	320	327	334	341	348
71	136	143	150	157	165	172	179	186	193	200	208	215	222	229	236	243	250	257	265	272	279	286	293	301	308	315	322	329	338	343	351	358
72	140	147	154	162	169	177	184	191	199	206	213	221	228	235	242	250	258	265	272	279	287	294	302	309	316	324	331	338	346	353	361	368
73	144	151	159	166	174	182	189	197	204	212	219	227	235	242	250	257	265	272	280	288	295	302	310	318	325	333	340	348	355	363	371	378
74	148	155	163	171	179	186	194	202	210	218	225	233	241	249	256	264	272	280	287	295	303	311	319	326	334	342	350	358	365	373	381	389
75	152	160	168	176	184	192	200	208	216	224	232	240	248	256	264	272	279	287	295	303	311	319	327	335	343	351	359	367	375	383	391	399
76	156	164	172	180	189	197	205	213	221	230	238	246	254	263	271	279	287	295	304	312	320	328	336	344	353	361	369	377	385	394	402	410

Obesity is very dangerous as it can lead to diabetes, high blood pressure, high cholesterol, stroke, cardiovascular disease, gallstones, gout, degenerative arthritis, and sleep apnea as well as other chronic illnesses. British researchers at the University of Oxford say that obesity can shorten your lifespan by 10 years, and raises the risk of heart disease, diabetes, kidney failure, lung failure, and cancer.[15]

Overeating and eating the wrong types of food are the leading causes of obesity as well as the lack of physical exercise. Fast food is so convenient for us yet all the fried food and sweets that we eat quickly lead to weight gain. Foods that contain refined carbohydrates, also called simple carbohydrates also lead to weight gain as the carbohydrates are absorbed quicker into the bloodstream and lead to a higher blood sugar level compared to eating foods that contain complex carbohydrates. Refer to Chapter X-Diet for more information.

Overeating is a nasty habit that is hard to break, I say this from experience. Overeating can be caused by many things, for me it was boredom. Sometimes I would find myself eating when I wasn't hungry, but I had nothing better to do. Binge eating can also be caused by sadness, anger, stress, or other emotional issues.

People who are physically inactive burn less calories than those who are physically active. I have heard many adults complain that children today are not as active as we were when we were young.

It is scary to see more and more children are becoming obese. Childhood obesity is becoming a very serious problem. Some schools in the US have started issuing fitness report cards showing the child's body mass index and grading the child's overall physical fitness. The readily available amount of unhealthy food is undermining the attempts at curbing childhood obesity, which is now the most common chronic medical condition facing children today.[16]

---

[15] Being Obese Can Shorten Life By Up To 10 Years, The Straits Times, March 19, 2009, Page A4.

[16] Fontanarosa, Phil B., MD, MBA< DeAngelis, Catherine D., MD, MPH, Wong, John E. L., MBBS, FACP. JAMA, National University Health System, Singapore, Host Diabetes, Obesity Meeting. JAMA The Journal of the American Medical Association. October 15, 2008. 1750-1751.

"Fast-food menus are a minefield of saturated fat, sugar, and extra calories . . ."

Diabetes, Vol. 14, No. 3, June/July 2009

Selected nutritional contents of popular food items:

Nutritional Information of Selected Popular Foods									
McDonalds									
	Calo-ries	Total Fat (g)	Satu-rated Fat (g)	Trans Fat (g)	Choles-terol (mg)	Sodium (mg)	Total Carbo-hydrates (g)	Sugars (g)	Protein (g)
Big Mac	540	29	10	1.5	75	1040	45	9	25
Quarter Pounder	410	19	7	1	65	730	37	8	24
Quarter Pounder w/Cheese	510	26	12	1.5	90	1190	40	9	29
Big 'N Tasty	460	24	8	1.5	70	720	37	8	24
Big 'N Tasty w/Cheese	510	28	11	1.5	85	960	38	8	27
Hamburger	250	9	3.5	0.5	25	520	31	6	12
Cheeseburger	300	12	6	0.5	40	750	33	6	15
McChicken	360	16	3	0	35	830	40	5	14
Premium Chicken Club Sandwich (crispy)	630	28	7	0.5	75	1420	60	13	36
Premium Chicken Club Sandwich (grilled)	530	17	6	0	90	1470	52	12	40
Fillet O Fish	380	18	3.5	0	40	640	38	5	15
Ranch Snack Wrap (crispy)	340	17	4.5	0	30	810	33	2	14
Ranch Snack Wrap (grilled)	270	10	4	0	45	830	26	2	18
Chicken Selects (3 piece)	400	24	3.5	0	50	1010	23	0	23
Chicken Selects (5 piece)	660	40	6	0	85	1680	39	0	38
Chicken McNuggets (6 piece)	280	17	3	0	40	600	16	0	10
Chicken McNuggets (10 piece)	460	29	5	0	70	1000	27	0	24
French Fries (small)	230	11	1.5	0	0	160	29	0	3
French Fries (medium)	380	19	2.5	0	0	270	48	0	4
French Fries (large)	500	25	3.5	0	0	350	63	0	6

Jack in the Box	Calo-ries	Total Fat (g)	Satu-rated Fat (g)	Trans Fat (g)	Choles-terol (mg)	Sodium (mg)	Total Carbo-hydrates (g)	Sugars (g)	Protein (g)
Sourdough Steak Melt	662	39	14	0	94	1484	39	2	36
Sirloin Cheeseburger	941	59	18	2	143	1890	60	11	40
Ultimate Cheeseburger	910	61	27	2	119	1493	52	9	37
Sourdough Jack	671	45	17	1	72	1174	39	6	24
Jumbo Jack	578	33	12	1	49	916	52	8	19
Jumbo Jack w/Cheese	660	39	16	1	72	1257	54	9	23
Big Cheeseburger	646	39	16	1	69	1147	51	8	23
Hamburger Deluxe	344	18	5	1	39	548	31	5	14
Chicken Sandwich	400	21	4.5	2.5	35	740	38	4	15
Jacks Spicy Chicken	550	24	6	3	50	1050	69	8	24
Sourdough Grilled Chicken Club	530	29	7	2	90	1440	34	5	36
French Fries (natural cut) (small)	290	15	3.5	4.5	0	540	35	1	4
French Fries (natural cut) (medium)	460	24	6	7	0	850	55	1	6
French Fries (natural cut) (large)	620	32	7	9	0	1150	75	1	9

Wendy's	Calo-ries	Total Fat (g)	Satu-rated Fat (g)	Trans Fat (g)	Choles-terol (mg)	Sodium (mg)	Total Carbo-hydrates (g)	Sugars (g)	Protein (g)
Triple w/everything and cheese	980	60	27	3.5	245	2010	43	9	69
Baconator	840	51	23	2.5	195	1880	38	8	56
Double w/everything and cheese	710	40	17	2	160	1440	41	9	47
Single w/everything	430	20	7	1	75	870	39	9	25
Jr. Bacon Cheeseburger	320	16	6	0.5	50	670	26	5	17
Jr. Cheeseburger Deluxe	300	14	6	0.5	45	730	29	7	15
Jr. Cheeseburger	270	11	5	0.5	40	690	27	6	15
Jr. Hamburger	230	8	3	0	30	490	27	5	13
Chicken Club Sandwich	540	25	8	0	75	1360	48	7	34
Ultimate Chicken Grill Sandwich	320	7	1.5	0	70	950	36	8	28
French Fries (small)	340	16	2.5	0	0	290	45	0	4
French Fries (medium)	430	20	3	0	0	370	56	0	6
French Fries (large)	550	26	4	0	0	480	72	0	7

	Calories	Total Fat (g)	Saturated Fat (g)	Trans Fat (g)	Cholesterol (mg)	Sodium (mg)	Total Carbohydrates (g)	Sugars (g)	Protein (g)
Chicken Nuggets (4 piece kids meal)	190	12	2	0	30	420	10	0	10
Chicken Nuggets (5 piece)	230	15	3	0	35	520	12	0	12
Chicken Nuggets (10 piece)	460	30	6	0	70	1040	24	0	24
Chocolate Frosty (small)	320	8	5	0	15	75	52	41	9
Chocolate Frosty (medium)	410	11	7	0.5	45	200	68	54	11
Chocolate Frosty (large)	530	14	9	0.5	55	260	86	69	14
Chili (small)	190	6	2.5	0	40	830	0.19	6	14
Chili (large)	280	9	3.5	0.5	60	1240	29	9	21

Hardees	Calories	Total Fat (g)	Saturated Fat (g)	Trans Fat (g)	Cholesterol (mg)	Sodium (mg)	Total Carbohydrates (g)	Sugars (g)	Protein (g)
Monster Burger	1060	79	29		185	1860	37		49
Bacon Double Cheeseburger	1000	70	25		185	1575	42		50
Bacon Cheeseburger	720	48	15		105	1200	42		30
Famous Star	510	35	10		80	860	41		24
Double Cheeseburger	480	28	13		75	1055	31		26
Cheeseburger	320	15	7		40	780	30		16
Hamburger	270	11	4		35	550	29		13
Grilled Chicken Sandwich	350	16	3		65	860	41		24
Chicken Fillet Sandwich	480	23	4		55	1190	44		24
Fishermans Fillet Sandwich	530	28	7		75	1280	45		25
French Fries (regular)	340	16	2		0	390	45		4
French Fries (large)	440	21	3		0	520	59		5
French Fries (monster)	510	24	3		0	590	67		6

Starbucks	Calories	Total Fat (g)	Saturated Fat (g)	Trans Fat (g)	Cholesterol (mg)	Sodium (mg)	Total Carbohydrates (g)	Sugars (g)	Protein (g)
Brewed Coffee (tall)	5	0	0	0	0	10	0	0	0
Cappuccino (nonfat milk) (tall)	60	0	0	0	15	70	9	0	8
Cappuccino (2% milk) (tall)	90	3.5	2	0	15	70	9	0	8
Caffe Latte (nonfat milk) (tall)	100	0	0	0	5	120	15	0	10
Caffe Latte (2% milk) (tall)	150	6	3.5	0	25	115	14	0	10
Vanilla Latte (nonfat milk) (tall)	150	0	0	0	5	115	28	27	9

Vanilla Latte (2% milk) (tall)	190	5	3.5	0	5	115	27	26	9
Caffe Mocha (nonfat milk) (tall)	170	2	0	0	5	100	32	25	10
Caffe Mocha (2% milk) (tall)	200	6	3.5	0	20	100	31	24	10
White Chocolate Mocha (nonfat milk) (tall)	270	4.5	3.5	0	5	190	47	45	12
White Chocolate Mocha (2% milk) (tall)	310	9	6	0	5	190	46	44	11
Strawberries & Crème Frappucino (tall)	290	1.5	0	0	5	210	60	53	8
Vanilla Bean Frappucino (tall)	260	2	0	0	5	230	53	44	9

A recent study published online in the Journal of the National Cancer Institute (June 26, 2009) found that people who ate a diet rich in fats were 36% more likely to contract pancreatic cancer. The risk of pancreatic cancer rises to 43% in those who consumed animal fats.

Chapter 13

Lifestyle Diet

"Eating right and being physically active aren't just a "diet" or a "program"—they are keys to a healthy lifestyle. With healthful habits, you may reduce your risk of many chronic diseases such as heart disease, diabetes, osteoporosis, and certain cancers, and increase your chances for a longer life."

> U.S. Department of Health and Human Services web site, Dietary Guidelines for Americans
> http://www.health.gov/DietaryGuidelines

The human body is more than a masterpiece of art. It is more than just our physical being, the Bible calls it the temple of the Holy Spirit. The human body is an intricately designed piece of machinery. Like all machinery, it operates on fuel, and like all machinery, the purer the fuel, the machinery operates at a higher level of efficiency. In the case of the human body, the fuel is food. To be more precise, it is the nutrients within the food we eat that fuels the body.

Today, not just in the United States, but throughout the world, the food that we consume contains much less than the nutrients required for our bodies to function at an optimum level. I am reminded of my Army days when someone put regular gasoline in my HUMVEE that had a diesel engine. Needless to say, after that, my HUMVEE did not operate properly. From then on, my Hummer went from 0 to 15 mph in about 3 minutes.

Likewise, when our bodies are fed improper food, they do not operate properly and the results can be disastrous. Our health is directly related to the fuel that we feed our bodies.

NUTRITION

Nutrition is the provision of the necessary materials (nutrients) needed to support the life of an organism, in this case, the human body.

The U.S. Department of Health and Human Services and the U.S. Department of Agriculture recommend 2 cups of fruits and 2 ½ cups of vegetables, particularly those high in fiber, and 3 cups each of whole grains and dairy. Saturated fats should be limited to 10% of the total number of calories per day and the total amount of fat consumed should be limited to 20-30% of total calories.[17] Sodium intake should be less than 2,300 mg per day. Persons with high blood pressure should limit sodium intake to less than 1,500 mg per day (keep in mind, a Big Mac has 1,040 mg of sodium).

I have heard amazing statistics that at least half of the population of the United States is on some kind of diet. The diet industry is a very lucrative industry to be in as is evident by all of the diet plans, weight loss pills and supplements on the market. More than 95% of people that loses weight while dieting will gain it back within 5 years. Clearly, losing weight and maintaining it at a healthy level is a lifelong goal. Instead of having quick diet mindset, we must have a lifestyle diet mindset. Our goal must be to live a long and healthy life.

A simple way to reduce weight is to reduce caloric intake. Depending on a persons body weight, adults need between 1200 and 2800 calories to maintain their average weight and meet the energy needs of their body. Generally, one pound equals 3500 calories. In other words, in order to lose one pound, you have to burn off 3500 more calories than you consume. It is extremely important not to deprive your body of essential vitamins and minerals when reducing caloric intake.

---

[17]   U.S. Department of Health and Human Services and U.S. Department of Agriculture. Dietary Guidelines for Americans 2005. Page 10.

Loosing fat will allow the cells of the body to absorb more glucose as they are designed to and the cells will respond properly to the insulin in the bloodstream.

Diet is linked to high blood pressure as well. Eating fruits and vegetables helps lower high blood pressure. The polyunsaturated fatty acid in plants and vegetables lower the risk of high blood pressure.[18] Prior to joining the Army, I had been a soda drinking carnivore. After going vegan, my blood pressure is consistently around 116/63. Prior to that, my blood pressure was dangerously high, consistently around 144/93, even though I was in fairly good shape and very active physically.

PROTEIN

Over the last decade or so high protein diets have been very popular. I've had several friends of mine proclaim that they will eat nothing but protein. Protein is essential for our bodies, however, we do not need large quantities of it. Our bodies only really need to intake 0.36 grams of protein for every pound that we weigh.[19]

FRUITS AND VEGETABLES

Fruits and veggies are the most important of all food groups. According to the US Department of Agriculture, eating a diet that is rich in fruits and vegetables may reduce the risk of diabetes, cardiovascular and coronary heart disease, stomach, mouth, and colon-rectum cancer, reduces the risk of developing kidney stones, and reduces the risk of bone loss. Diets rich in fruits and vegetables naturally help reduce blood pressure and blood cholesterol levels, and reduces the risk of stroke.

---

[18]   China Daily, In Brief, page 19. Veggies Help Keep BP in Check. September 10, 2008.

[19]   Food and Nutrition Board, Institute of Medicine. *Dietary Reference intakes for Energy, Carbohydrate, Fiber, Bat, Fatty Acids, Cholesterol, Protein, and Amino Acids.* Washington, DC: National Academy Press, 2002.

Fruits and vegetables naturally contains vitamins and minerals. Most fruits and vegetables are naturally low in fat and calories. Not one fruit or vegetable contains cholesterol.

Over the years, before becoming a vegan, there were times where I would eat only fruits and vegetables for a day or two at a time, without even giving it much thought. I did notice, however, that on those occasions I did seem to have a lot more energy and generally felt better overall. Each of those occasions reminded me of the story in the Bible of Shadrak, Meshak, and Abednego, whose countenances were much fairer than everyone else's when they ate only vegetables instead of the king's meat.

GRAINS

Whole grains—The US Department of Agriculture recommends that teen and adult men consume about 7 ounces of grains per day and teen and adult women should consume about 6 ounces of grains. Grains are rice, oats, cornmeal, barley, etc. and are very beneficial when eaten as a whole grain. Whole grain fiber reduces blood cholesterol levels, lowers the risk of heart disease, increases bowel movement, and most beneficial of all, whole grain fiber gives you a feeling of fullness with less calories. Whole grains are essential in building healthy bone tissue and protecting cells from oxidation. Read the food labels carefully to make sure that you are actually getting whole grains.

> "Foods labeled with the words 'multi-grain,' stone-ground,' '100% wheat,' 'cracked wheat,' 'seven-grain,' or 'bran' are usually not whole-grain products.'
> MyPyramid.gov (US Department of Agriculture)

The B vitamins in the whole grains are essential in the body's metabolism, assisting in the conversion of fats, carbohydrates, and protein into energy for the body to use. The B vitamins in whole grains are essential to the healthy function of the nervous system. Folic acid, a B vitamin is also essential in the forming of red blood cells, and iron is used to carry oxygen in the bloodstream.

Refined grains—Advertisers tout the words "refined," "fortified," and "enriched" in commercials and food packaging to get our attention and to get us to buy their products and to make us think that their products are healthier than the others on the shelf. Refined grains have had their bran and germ stripped in order to give them a longer shelf life. More about refined grains under "carbohydrates."

CARBOHYDRATES

The recommended intake of carbohydrates is 14 grams per 1,000 calories. Many dietitians are critical of diets that are high in carbohydrates as the carbohydrates get broken down into sugar during digestion, thereby increasing the glucose levels in the bloodstream. There is, however, a difference between complex carbohydrates and processed carbohydrates. The processed carbohydrates, also called simple carbohydrates and refined carbohydrates, come from processed food such as refined sugar, rice, flour, etc. The processed carbohydrates have a higher glycemic index than natural carbohydrates because they have lost a lot of their nutrients and fiber during the processing. The refined carbohydrates greatly increase blood sugar levels as they remain in the digestive tract longer and release glucose into the blood stream.

Carbohydrates are the sugars, starches, and fiber that are found in fruits, vegetables, and grains. Carbohydrates are also found in milk. Carbohydrates are very important as they are converted to glucose to supply energy for the body. The fiber, however, does not get converted into glucose.

The complex carbohydrates are naturally present in fruits and vegetables. The complex carbohydrates pass through the digestive system before the carbohydrates can be converted into sugar. That is the general rule of thumb regarding carbohydrates, however it is important to also consider the fact that the body processes carbohydrates from both groups differently. According to the U.S. Department of health and the U.S.D.A., "diets rich in dietary fiber have been shown to have a number of beneficial effects."[20] Keeping

---

[20]   U.S. Department of Health and Human Services and U.S. Department of Agriculture. Dietary Guidelines for Americans 2005. Page 47.

this in mind, it is important to avoid foods and beverages that are high in added sugars.

> "Whole-grain or high-fiber carb food-whole-grain bread, brown rice, and lentils, for example-break down more slowly in your body than do simple-carb foods like doughnuts, white bread, and cookies. These more complex carbs also provide a steady stream of energy."
>
> Diabetes, vol.14, No. 3, June/July 2009

The author of this quote warns readers not to eat these complex carbs in large quantities. The important thing to notice is that the complex carbohydrates do not get processed into glucose as fast as the refined carbohydrates.

THE VEGAN DIET

The one diet that has consistently proven to lower blood pressure, lower cholesterol, help with weight control, reverse cardiovascular disease, reverse diabetes, and help people overcome many adverse health issues is the all natural vegan diet. Speaking from my own personal experience and the experience I have witnessed in others, it is amazing to see the difference diet can make.

The biggest misnomer concerning the vegan diet is that many think that people cannot get enough protein by eating a plant based diet. The fact is, vegans get plenty of protein in their diet, in spite of the emphasis placed on high protein diets these days. As mentioned earlier, the average adult needs only about .36 grams of protein per pound per day. A 200 pound man only needs 72 grams of protein per day. Vegetables, legumes, grains, and nuts contain more protein than a lot of people realize. Amino acids are the building blocks of protein. Of the twenty common amino acids, the human body is only able to produce eleven of them, therefore we must obtain the other nine amino acids through our diet.

What makes the vegan diet the healthiest diet of all is the fact that it contains less fat, saturated fat and calories than meat-based diets, and above all, the vegan diet contains no cholesterol. Since foods that are high in fat contribute to diabetes and other diseases, the vegan lifestyle diet lowers glucose levels and contributes to weight loss and leads to overall better health by actually reversing the process that leads to these diseases.

Opponents to the vegan diet are concerned with omega-3 and omega-6 fatty acids. Most are convinced that the only source of omega-3 and omega-6 fatty acids are contained in fish. This is untrue as these fatty acids are also present in leafy green vegetables, legumes, soybeans, flaxseed, and wheat germ. The downside of obtaining these essential fatty acids from fish is the presence of mercury and other toxins that are found in fish along with saturated fat and cholesterol.

In my case, arthritis, sarcoidosis, diabetes, and lupus all cleared up within 3 months of turning to the vegan lifestyle diet. It makes sense that since the food we eat is gradually deteriorating our bodies, turning around and eating a perfectly healthy diet would turn things around for the better, the body is notorious for healing itself when it is treated right. In the book, "The Lupus Recovery Diet," author Jill Harrington describes how she and many others, including myself, have recovered from diseases such as lupus, rheumatoid arthritis, fibromyalgia, sarcoidosis, and diabetes, simply by adopting a new lifestyle diet.

UN-SUPERSIZE ME

The documentary "Supersize Me" came out several years ago, causing a stir and an awareness of the affects of today's modern fast food. The movie followed Morgan Spurlock as he ate at McDonald's 3 times a day, every day for a month. He sampled everything on the menu at least once, and if asked if he wanted his meal supersized, he had to say yes. The movie chronicled the affects it had on his health. During the one-month experiment, he consumed about 5,000 calories per day, gaining 24 ½ pounds during that time and gaining a 13% body mass increase. The movie also mentioned that the all fast-food diet caused erectile dysfunction.

When I started eating vegan, I experienced the exact opposite side-effects. The first month of being vegan, I had lost about 31 pounds, my blood pressure dropped and stabilized to a perfect 116/63. In regards to libido, let me just say that if every man went on a vegan diet, I am positive that there would be absolutely no need for Viagra or any other male enhancement medication. This is due to the increase in blood flow throughout the body that the vegan diet promotes.

There are many critics of the Supersize Me documentary, saying that there is no one on earth that eats at McDonald's 3 times a day, every day of the week, but that does not change the fact that fast-food in general is very unhealthy.

LONGER LIFE

According to a study at Loma Linda University, vegans live on average about 15 years longer than people who eat meat. Vegetarians (those that consume some refined foods and dairy products) live about 7 years longer than people who eat meat. The China Health Project concluded that Chinese people that consume the least amount of fat and animal products are the least likely to contract cancer, heart disease, and other degenerative diseases.

OVERCOMING DIABETES

"Diabetes is not necessarily a one-way street. Early studies suggest that persons with type 2 diabetes can improve and, in some cases, even reverse the disease by switching to an unrefined, vegan diet."

Andrew Nicholson, M.D.,
Diabetes: Can a Vegan Diet Reverse Diabetes?

As many have gratefully found out, including myself, diabetes is completely reversible. Just as obesity and the consumption of fats and refined sugars in our American diet has lead to the epidemic of diabetes, the naturally low-fat vegan diet has led to the complete reversal of diabetes. The cells become less and less saturated with fat and glucose and the body naturally metabolizes glucose as it was intended to.

Many studies have shown that the vegan diet has greatly improved, if not completely reversed diabetes altogether. The Reversing Diabetes program offered by the Weimar Institute has helped many diabetics overcome diabetes and get off of all diabetes medication. Unfortunately, studies and programs like these do not get much recognition in the media.

RELIEF FOR OSTEOARTHRITIS SUFFERERS

A major benefit of the vegan diet is weight loss. As previously mentioned, obesity is one of the causes of osteoarthritis, putting unnecessary pressure and weight on joints. Inflammation and deterioration of cartilage causes pain and immobility. The vegan diet naturally reduces inflammation throughout the body and has been found to naturally lubricate the joints, reversing the deterioration of the naturally occurring lubricating cartilage in the joints.

For more information, I encourage you to read more at the NEWSTART website at *http://www.newstart.com/disorder.php?action=osteoarthritis.*

RELIEF FOR PEOPLE WITH AUTOIMMUNE DISEASES
(Lupus, Sarcoidosis, Rheumatoid Arthritis, etc.)

People suffering from autoimmune diseases should be glad to know that a vegan diet is naturally anti-inflammatory. The vegan diet boosts levels of natural antibodies that help fight against rheumatoid arthritis. The natural antioxidants help the body to eliminate the chemicals in our bodies that causes inflammation. There are reports of rheumatoid arthritis sufferers completely overcoming arthritis by eliminating dairy products from their diet. Many others have reported complete victory over rheumatoid arthritis simply by changing their diet.[21]

Researchers in Stockholm, Sweden have concluded that a gluten-free vegan diet raises the levels of natural antibodies that fight the compounds

---

[21]   Skoldstam L. Fasting and vegan diet in rheumatoid arthritis. Scand J Rheumatol 1986;15:219-23

6. McDougall J, Bruce B, Spiller G, Westerdahl J, McDougall M. Effects of a very low-fat, vegan diet in subjects with rheumatoid arthritis. J Altern Complement Med. 2002 Feb;8(1):71-5.

7. Hafstrom I, Ringertz B, Spangberg A, von Zweigbergk L, Brannemark S, Nylander I, Ronnelid J, Laasonen L, Klareskog L. A vegan diet free of gluten improves the signs and symptoms of rheumatoid arthritis: the effects on arthritis correlate with a reduction in antibodies to food antigens. Rheumatology (Oxford). 2001 Oct;40(10):1175-9.

that cause the inflammatory symptoms of rheumatoid arthritis as reported by the United Press International, March 19, 2008.

> "Rheumatoid arthritis (RA) patients who eat a gluten-free vegan diet could be better protected against heart attacks and stroke. RA is a major risk factor for these cardiovascular diseases, but a gluten-free vegan diet was shown to lower cholesterol, low-density lipoprotein (LDL) and oxidizedLDL (OxLDL), as well as raising the levels of natural antibodies against the damaging compounds in the body that cause symptoms of the chronic inflammatory disease rheumatoid arthritis, such as phosphorylcholine."
>
> Science Daily (Mar. 20, 2008)

Just like in rheumatoid arthritis, the vegan diet raises the level of natural antibodies that fight against autoimmune diseases. The vegan diet has natural anti-inflammatory effects on the body's tissues, countering the inflammation that occurs when the immune system attacks the body.

For more information, I strongly encourage you to read more at the NEWSTART website at http://www.newstart.com/disorder.php?action=rheumatoid_arthritis.

OBESITY

For more information and testimonials on how the vegan diet can bring your weight to normal levels, refer to http://www.newstart.com/disorder.php?action=obesity.

Chapter 14

Exercise

The key to losing weight is to burn off more calories than you consume. All types of physical activity burns some amount of calories. The duration and intensity of the physical activity will determine the amount of calories burned during the session of exercise. A regular exercise routine along with a healthy diet is key to reaching and maintaining a healthy weight, leading to a long and healthy life. Just as obesity is a major cause of diabetes, weight loss is a sure-fire way of lowering blood glucose levels or even eliminating diabetes altogether. The U.S. Department of Health and Human Services and the U.S. Department of Agriculture recommend 30 minutes of exercise in addition to normal daily activity on "most days of the week," in order to lower the risk of chronic diseases in adults.[22] In order to maintain or loose weight, it is recommended to exercise 60-90 minutes with a mixture of stretching, cardiovascular, and resistance exercises on a regular basis.

Not only does exercise burn excess fat, it lowers blood sugar levels to a healthier level, lowers blood pressure, reduces the risk of cardiovascular disease and increases the levels of good HDL cholesterol. Exercise also helps the body's tissues respond to insulin, lowering blood glucose levels.[23]

---

[22] U.S. Department of Health and Human Services and U.S. Department of Agriculture. Dietary Guidelines for Americans 2005. Page 10.

[23] Ober, Patrick, M.D. How Important Is Regular Exercise For Type 1 and Type 2 Diabetes? ABC News. January 11, 2008.

Exercise also reduces the amount of fat around the liver, lowering the risk of fatty liver disease.

During exercise, muscles contract and relax off and on. This action of movement in the muscles burn glucose as energy, even without the use of insulin. Exercise increases the body's sensitivity to insulin, causing the body to need less insulin to process the glucose in the bloodstream. Exercise not only burns calories, it also increases the body's metabolism. As we exercise, our heart beats faster and blood flow is increased throughout the body, making the heart stronger and reduces the risk of heart disease. Exercise also helps the body to use the natural insulin more effectively and efficiently.

Exercise may be very difficult at first, however, the more that we exercise, the easier it gets. It is easier to begin lightly and gradually work to more strenuous workouts.

Always consult with your doctor prior to starting any exercise program. I would always recommend beginning any exercise regimen with a professional trainer also. Most health clubs have professional trainers on staff.

Recent study is being conducted regarding genetic variations that make some people more susceptible to weight gain. While this may be true, it should not be used as an excuse for becoming overweight. In any case, physical activity will reverse the effects of the genetic variant.[24]

A recent study shows that a regular weight lifting regimen increases the levels of free testosterone.

---

[24]   China Daily, Life Health. Daily DIY Guide To Getting Fit For Those With The Fat Factor. September 10, 2008, page 19.

Chapter 15

The Chemicals We Put Into Our Bodies

"Life is like a sewer, what you get out of it depends on what you put into it."

Tom Leher, "An Evening Wasted with Tom Leher"

"American fastfood, what a stupid way to die."

Randy Stonehill, "American Fastfood."

The same can be said about our bodies. Those who are in good shape are that way because of diet and exercise. Those of us who are obese or are in poor shape are that way because of poor diet and/or lack of exercise. We must realize that we have the body that we have because we have worked for it. Some people eat right and exercise regularly and are in good physical condition. Others of us eat poorly and don't get enough exercise and are in poor physical condition. We should never be surprised at how good or bad we look physically.

A lot of people joke about the fact that nearly everything in food causes cancer these days. I've heard people joke about it for many years. That seems to be the way we deal with many things that we don't want to face. It is easier to ignore the warnings and joke about them than it is to acknowledge them. It is not a joke, cancer has been increasing at an alarming rate in this country.

Everything we eat has an effect on our bodies. On one hand, if we eat healthy and eat food rich in nutrition, our bodies absorb the nutrients and awards us with good health. When we eat foods that are full of chemicals and fats, our bodies pay us back with ill health and problems. Read the labels carefully of the foods you eat and take note. Ask yourself and ask your doctor which foods you should eat:

Acrylamide: has been found to cause cancer in animals and is found in many American food products.

Ascorbic acid: Another name for vitamin C and is an antioxidant. Side effects include upset stomach, diarrhea, frequent urination, and mouth sores. Kidney stones may also develop with larger doses.

Aspartame: A popular artificial sweetener found and found in many foods, drinks, and medicines ingested everyday. Ingestion of aspartame causes Formaldehyde Accumulation inside the body. Aspartame has been linked to leukemia, lymphoma, and cancer in laboratory rats.[25]T Aspartame has also been linked to weight gain, memory loss and brain tumors.

BHA (Butylated hydroxyanisole) and **BHT** (butylated hydroxytoluene): Used to preserve fats and oils. BHA and BHT has been link to cancer in rats.

Food coloring: Some food colorings are carcinogenic and may also cause hyperactivity, allergies, and learning difficulties.

High fructose corn syrup: Produced by the processing of corn starch into glucose, which is then processed into fructose. Enzymes used in this processed are genetically modified to make them stable. Laboratory rats given fructose developed anemia, high cholesterol, and heart hypertrophy (enlarging of the heart enlarged until it explodes).

Hydrogenated oils: Hydrogenated and partially hydrogenated oils contain high levels of trans fat and lead to obesity as it does not satisfy

---

[25]   SCIENCE VOL 317 6 JULY 2007 page 31 Souring on Fake Sugar

your sense of hunger (they do not satisfy the body's need for essential fatty acids). There is a link between multiple sclerosis, allergies and arthritis and hydrogenated oils. Hydrogenated oils can create trans fats, leading to cardiovascular disease and diabetes.

MSG (Monosodium Glutamate): MSG is a food additive used to enhance flavor and is found in many foods. Controversy abounds as the FDA maintains that MSG is safe for consumption (with short term allergies in some people), while others claim that MSG is responsible for obesity, Alzheimer's disease, and other diseases.

Nitrates and nitrites: Often found in preserved meats, nitrates and nitrites can form nitrosamines, a compound that has been linked to cancer in laboratory animals.

Phosphoric acid: A colourless liquid, used in the manufacture of fertilizers, detergents and pharmaceuticals and as an additive in cola drinks. Phosphoric acid causes the erosion of tooth enamel and can even cause deterioration to your bones.[26] Phosphoric acid is used to remove rust from steel.

Polyunsaturated fat: an essential fatty acid mostly found in fruits and vegetables; important in the management of heart disease.

Potassium Bromate: Used in bread products, bromate has been linked to cancer in laboratory animals.

Propyl Gallate: This preservative, used to prevent fats and oils from spoiling, might cause cancer. Often used with BHA and BHT.

Saturated fat: A type of fat found in greatest amounts in sources of foods from animals and a few plants. These foods can contribute to

---

[26] http://www.naturalnews.com/021774.html Phosphoric acid in sodas nearly as damaging to teeth as battery acid. Thursday, April 05, 2007 by: NaturalNews staff, citizen journalist

cardiovascular disease, high cholesterol, and the development of some cancers.

Sodium: High sodium levels in the bloodstream can lead to high blood pressure and kidney disease and also depletes the body of potassium and may lead to cancer.

Sodium Benzoate: A preservative used in some soft drinks. When mixed with the vitamin C additive in soft drinks it forms a carcinogen called benzene.

Sulfites: May cause allergic reaction, headaches, nausea, and diarrhea.

TBHQ (tertiary butylhydroquinone): A preservative made of fats and oils. Controversy surrounds the use of this preservative as some have claimed that it can cause nausea and vomiting and even death if consumed in high enough quantities.

Chapter 16

Additional Testimonials

Many others have overcome diabetes, arthritis, autoimmune diseases, obesity, and other medical problems, and enriched their lives by switching to a natural vegan diet.

Qin Tianfu, Qingzhou, China

I joined the Army right out of high school, and after serving in the Army for 15 years I moved with my family back to my hometown of Qingzhou, China. I continued to work for the government until Qingzhou got its own newspaper, where I went to work as its first editor-in-chief. I worked at the newspaper for 10 years until I retired at the age of 60. I've always enjoyed writing and often wrote articles for various newspapers throughout China. After retiring from the newspaper I was able to edit two books for publication.

I had always been in good health, however, after retiring, I gained some weight and my blood pressure began to creep up. In July, 2007, I noticed what's called black eye floaters, tiny black specs in my eyes. I saw the doctor and he told me that my eyes just needed some rest and told me to go home. A week later I began to feel very week and had to go to the bathroom very often throughout the day and especially at night. Three days later I was too weak to even stand up and was immediately admitted to the hospital. The doctors told me that my blood pressure and blood sugar levels were very high and started me on oral medications. After three days of taking medications in the hospital my blood sugar level was still too high and the doctors wanted me to begin taking insulin. I dreaded taking insulin because my doctor told me that once I started taking insulin I would have to take it for the rest of my life. My doctor warned me that if I did not get my blood sugar level back to normal it could result in kidney damage, so I agreed to take insulin. After a few days of taking insulin, my blood sugar dropped to normal and the doctor put me back on oral medications and stopped the insulin. The doctor ordered me to walk 1km per day and to stop eating meat and refined flour, sugar, and grains. After 6 months, I went back to the hospital for a checkup. My regular doctor was out so another doctor saw me. He asked me why I was there and I told him it was because of diabetes. The doctor checked my blood sugar and told me that there was no sign of ever having diabetes. The doctor was shocked when he saw my records and found that I used to be a diabetic but no longer have diabetes. The doctor told me that he had never seen diabetes cured by diet and exercise without medication. I had been told by my previous doctor that I would always be diabetic and would have to rely on insulin injections the rest of my life. I am happy that today I am perfectly healthy without having to take any medications.

Robert Forster, San Antonio, Texas

I've spent almost all of my life in the beautiful city of San Antonio. In high school I played football and ran track. I was in very good shape up through my college days. As I entered the work force as a computer programmer I got into the habit of eating fast food a few times a week. I thought that as long as I still went to the gym regularly the fast food would not harm me. As the years passed by, I ate out more and more often and gradually put on a lot of weight. I started my own business and found that I did not have the amount of free time that I used to have and began to eat out almost all the time. By the time I reached 40 I weighed 270 pounds. I noticed my vision getting blurry and just thought it was due to my prescription changing and got a new prescription for my glasses. After about a month, I noticed that my vision becoming blurry again. I thought it was because of the long hours that I was putting in at the office.

I went back to the optometrist to get my vision rechecked. The optometrist told me that before I spend more money on new glasses I should talk to my doctor and get my blood sugar checked. He told me that diabetes can cause blurry vision and can lead to more serious trouble if it goes unchecked. Due to my hectic schedule I didn't make an appointment with my doctor for another couple of months. I also noticed that I had to urinate rather frequently, which is another symptom of diabetes according to the information that my optometrist gave me.

I eventually went to see my doctor and he diagnosed me with diabetes, my blood sugar level was 481. He told me that I would have to take insulin for the rest of my life. After taking my initial injections of insulin I decided that I would do whatever I had to do to get my blood sugar back to normal so that I would not have to take insulin anymore.

My mother is a vegan and in excellent health and told me about someone in her church that reversed diabetes by becoming a vegan and exercising regularly. My mom set up a meeting with this man who's name is Tim, the next weekend. Tim showed me a bunch of documentation that he had collected regarding the effects of a vegan diet and exercise on diabetes. He shared with me the recipes that he had collected and helped me on my way. We met daily to walk around the neighborhood and in the park and we even met to cook together. I am 49 years old now and am in excellent shape, many people now tell me that I look 10-15 years younger than I actually am and have more energy now than I did when I was in my mid-thirties.

For additional testimonials, refer to the following:

The Lupus Recovery Diet, by Jill Harrington
http://www.newstart.com/success_stories.php
http://www.reversingdiabetes.org/Testimonials.aspx
http://www.drmcdougall.com/star.html

A Note To The Critics

There are many critics of the vegan diet and many more are doubtful of its benefits, particularly when it comes to testimonials such as mine. I myself thought it laughable that my health condition could be cured, and cured so easily at that.

To the critics and nay-sayers I say this: don't knock it until you've tried it. Before discrediting the vegan diet, try it for three weeks and notice the health benefits for yourself. As I mentioned before, I actually went on the vegan diet accidentally, I was looking for an alternative to prednisone, I had no intention of becoming a vegan. My health turned around quickly and dramatically as many others have experienced for themselves.

IT REALLY WORKS.

Recipes

Here are some very easy recipes to help get started cooking vegan. Remember, when I first started, I made a lot of mistakes and found that the easier the better.

Guacamole

INGREDIENTS:

3 Avocados, very ripe (black and soft)
½ chopped onion
1 chopped tomato
½ chopped green pepper
1 chopped jalapeno (optional)
¼ lime
¼ lemon
1 tsp salt
1 tsp pepper
1 tsp chili powder
1 tsp ground cumin
1 tsp ground coriander

1. Cut the avocados in half and spoon out the seed. Save the seed for later.
2. Place avocados into mixing bowl and mash with a fork.
3. Add the rest of the ingredients and stir thoroughly.
4. Add salt, pepper, and chili powder to taste.
Serve with tortilla chips or alongside other recipes.

Black Bean Vegan Veggie Burger:

INGREDIENTS:

½ diced onion
½ thinly sliced green peppers, no more than ¼-inch long
1 can black beans, drain well
½ cup flour
2 slices crumbled bread
2 tsp beef flavoring
1 tsp onion powder
1 tsp garlic powder
½ tsp salt
½ tsp pepper

1. Sautee onions, peppers and tomatoes no more than 5 minutes.
2. Completely mash black beans.
3. Mix ingredients together until thoroughly mixed.

Form into patties about ½-inch thick and place on broiler and broil 3-5 minutes on each side. Be careful not to burn patties. Patties will not be firm enough for the grill. Veggie burgers may also be fried in a frying pan. I use a small amount of water instead of oil or non-stick spray.

Lentil Vegan Veggie Burger:

INGREDIENTS:

¼ diced onion
¼ thinly sliced green peppers, no more than ¼-inch long
¼ cup finely grated carrots
3 cups cooked lentils
¾ cup bread crumbs
¼ cup water
2 tsp beef flavoring

2 tsp chopped parsley
3 tbsp tomato paste
½ tsp salt
½ tsp pepper

1. Sautee onions, peppers and tomatoes until tender.
2. Completely mash lentils.
3. Mix ingredients together until thoroughly mixed.

Form into patties about ½-inch thick and place on broiler and broil 3-5 minutes on each side. Be careful not to burn patties. Patties will not be firm enough for the grill. Veggie burgers may also be fried in a frying pan until thoroughly heated and browned on each side. I use a small amount of water instead of oil or non-stick spray.

Black beans and rice

INGREDIENTS:

½ green pepper
½ red pepper
¼ onion
½ tomato
3 cups black beans
1 cup brown rice (uncooked)
1 tsp salt
1 tsp pepper
1 tsp ground cumin
1 clove garlic (optional)

1. Chop the green and red pepper, onion, garlic, and tomato into small pieces (I prefer cutting them into tiny slivers).
2. Prepare and cook black beans per instructions on package.
3. Cook brown rice per instructions on package.

4. Sautee peppers, onion, tomato and garlic in frying pan with small amount of water (enough to keep ingredients from sticking. Add additional water as necessary.
5. Remove about half of the black beans and put in a blender. Blend for 5 seconds or until beans have reached desired consistency and pour back into pot with the rest of the beans and continue to cook.
6. Add peppers, onion, tomato and garlic to black beans and continue to cook until beans are fully cooked.
7. Add cumin and salt and pepper to taste.

Place cooked rice on serving dish. Cover rice with black beans and serve.

OPTIONS:

1. Make artificial cheese spread, warm in saucepan and pour on top of black beans.
2. Crumble organic whole grain tortilla chips and spread over black beans.

Pinto beans and rice

INGREDIENTS:

½ green pepper
½ red pepper
1 jalapeno pepper (optional)
¼ onion
½ tomato
3 cups pinto beans
1 cup brown rice (uncooked)
1 tsp salt
1 tsp pepper
1 tsp ground cumin

1. Chop the green and red pepper, jalapeno pepper, onion, garlic, and tomato into small slivers.

2. Prepare and cook pinto beans per instructions on package.
3. Cook brown rice per instructions on package.
4. Sautee peppers, onion, tomato and garlic in frying pan with small amount of water (enough to keep ingredients from sticking. Add additional water as necessary.
5. Remove a little less than half of the pinto beans and put in a blender. Blend for 5 seconds or until beans have reached desired consistency and pour back into pot with the rest of the beans and continue to cook.
6. Add peppers, onion, tomato and garlic to pinto beans and continue to cook until beans are fully cooked.
7. Add cumin and salt and pepper to taste.

Can be served in several different ways:

1. Mix beans and rice together and serve as a side dish.
2. Mix beans and rice together and serve as a bean & rice burrito in whole grain tortillas. Goes great with guacamole and salsa.
3. Place cooked rice on serving dish and cover with beans.

Arroz con Pollo (Rice and Chicken)

Arroz con pollo is a very popular and tasty dish in Mexico. This recipe replaces the chicken with soy curls.

INGREDIENTS:

1 green pepper
1 red pepper
1/2 onion
½ tomato
2 cups brown rice (uncooked)
1 cup soy curls. Can be substituted with vegan chicken breast fillets cut into slices.
3 tsp Chicnish seasoning
2 tsp salt

2 tsp pepper
1 tsp ground cumin
2 tsp cilantro
1 tsp cayenne pepper
1 clove garlic (optional)

1. Chop the green and red pepper, onion, garlic, and tomato into ½-inch by 1-inch pieces.
2. Soak soy curls in warm water for 15 minutes until tender.
3. Cook brown rice per instructions on package.
4. Sautee peppers, onion, tomato in frying pan with small amount of water (enough to keep ingredients from sticking. Add additional water as necessary.
5. Add soy curls to frying pan and cook with peppers, tomato and onions on medium for 3-5 minutes, stirring constantly. Add chicnish seasoning, cumin, salt and pepper to taste.
6. Add rice to frying pan and stir ingredients on medium for 1 minute.

Serve with chips and salsa and whole grain tortillas. Guacamole and sour supreme (soy sour cream) go well on the side.

Stir fry

You can't go wrong with this one. The best part is, you can add or subtract anything you want to and as many or little veggies you want (the more the better), this is a recipe that you can continually experiment with.

INGREDIENTS:

1 cup of spinach
½ cup shredded cabbage
½ cup shredded carrots
¼ cup of bean sprouts
½ cup broccoli
½ cup corn or baby corn

3 tsp Liquid Aminos
2 cups brown rice (uncooked)
1 tsp pepper
1 tsp salt
1 tsp ground cumin

1. Cook the brown rice per instructions on package.
2. Warm up frying pan, using small amount of water, add vegetables, stirring constantly on medium low for 5 minutes.
3. Add brown rice and liquid aminos to frying pan and stir. Add salt, pepper, and cumin.

Serve on individual plates or eat directly out of the frying pan like I do.

Roasted Veggies

INGREDIENTS:

1 cup of spinach
½ cup shredded cabbage
½ cup shredded carrots
¼ cup of bean sprouts
½ cup broccoli
½ cup corn or baby corn
¼ cup green beans
1 potato
2 cups brown rice (uncooked)
2 tsp pepper
2 tsp salt
1 tsp ground cumin
3 tsp chili powder

1. Cut the potato into ½-inch cubes and boil until cooked.
2. Place all veggies, including cooked potatoes in a gallon sized zip-lock bag. Place pepper, salt, cumin, and chili powder and mix into cup of water.

3. Pour water mixture into zip-locked bag and mix thoroughly until veggies are covered with spices.
4. Place veggies into baking dish and bake for 1-hour at 350 degrees.
5. Cook brown rice per instructions on package.

Place rice on serving dish and cover with roasted veggies. (Option) Mix rice and veggies together and serve.

Vegetable Radiatore Alfredo

My favorite: Vegan Wayne's World Vegetable Radiatore recipe that works. You don't have to make this while watching Waynes World, but it is more fun that way. This is the first recipe that I made that actually turned out right.

INGREDIENTS:

1 cup water
3/4 cup cashews
1 teaspoon salt (well, however much you want)
2 tablespoons food yeast
2 cloves garlic (or some minced garlic)
1 shallot (I just found out what that is too)
1 teaspoon onion powder
1 tablespoon & 1 teaspoon Liquid Aminos (optional, I didn't use it)
1/2 cup soy milk (optional, I didn't use it either, I forgot)
1/4 cup finely chopped parsley
1/2 cup Soy Curls (optional), can be substituted with vegan chicken breast fillets, cut into strips.
1 1/2 cup Pico De Gallo (finely chopped onion, tomato, green & red pepper-equal amounts of each)
1/4 cup Oregano (optional)
1/4 cup Italian Seasoning (optional)
3 Tablespoons Vegan Parmesan Cheese Substitute

1. Put the movie "Wayne's World" in the VCR and push play. Turn up loud enough to hear it in the kitchen.
2. Blend 1 cup water with cashews, salt, food yeast, garlic, shallot and onion powder to process until very smooth and creamy. Add another cup of water, liquid aminos and milk if you want to, but you'd better have a bigger skillet than mine.
3. Soak soy curls in hot tap water for 15 minutes.
4. Boil enough water to cook the pasta (but don't watch it, it won't boil if you do). Throw in the pasta for 5 minutes
5. Throw the Pico De Gallo into a skillet and marinate with Parsley, Oregano and Italian Seasoning.
6. Add the Alfredo Sauce from the blender to the Pico De Gallo along with Vegan Parmesan Cheese Substitute.
7. Add cooked pasta and soy curls to the mix. Hopefully, your skillet will hold it all, mine did just barely.
8. Put it all in a plate and go into the living room to watch the rest of "Wayne's World," it should be at the part where Wayne and Garth drive to Milwaukee to see Alice Cooper.

Potato Soup

1 cup finely chopped onion
1 cup finely chopped celery
4-6 peeled, cubed potatoes
4 cups soy milk
½ cup soy sour cream
2 tbs Earth Balance Margarine
1 tsp dill weed
2 tsp salt
2 tsp pepper

1. Combine onion, celery, potatoes, salt, and pepper together in a pot, cover with enough water to cook.
2. Mash potatoes when they are cooked and place back into the pot.

3. Add soy milk, soy sour cream, margarine and dill weed and cook an additional 5 minutes.

Vegan Corn Chowder

INGREDIENTS

1 small onion chopped
1 cup chopped carrots
1 cup chopped celery
2 cups corn
2 cubes vegetable bouillon
2 cups soy milk
1 tbs flour
1 tsp dried parsley
1 tsp garlic powder
1 tsp salt
1 tsp pepper

1. Sautee onions, celery, carrots and garlic powder.
2. Bring a pot of water to a boil over high heat. Add bouillon cubes.
3. Reduce heat to medium and add all other ingredients except soy milk when bouillon cubes have dissolved.
4. When vegetables are tender, reduce heat to low and add 1 cup soy milk.
5. Add second cup of soy milk and flour. Add parsley, salt and pepper.
6. Stir constantly for 15-20 minutes until chowder thickens.

Glossary

Acidosis Abnormally high acidic level in the bloodstream.

Addison's disease A hormone deficiency caused by damage to the adrenal glands. Symptoms include weakness, loss of weight, and low blood pressure.

Adrenal glands Two small organs near the kidneys that release hormones which control metabolism, fluid balance, and blood pressure.

Amyotrophy Progressive wasting and atrophy of muscle tissues. Diabetics experience the wasting of the thigh muscles.

Angina Chest pain due to reduced blood flow and oxygen to the heart.

Antibodies Specialized proteins created by the white blood cells in response to the presence of antigens in the body.

Antigen A foreign substance that can trigger an immune response, resulting in production of an antibody as a part of the body's defense.

Antinuclear antibody test (ANA) is a test for autoimmune disorders. It tests for antibodies that are directed against the nucleus of the body's cells.

Artery Arteries are blood vessels that carry blood away from the heart.

Atherosclerosis The process in which plaque builds up in the inner lining of an artery.

Arthritis is a painful Inflammation of the joints which causes stiffness and limitation of movement.

Autoimmune diseases are types of diseases in which the body's immune system malfunctions and attacks the body's own tissues.

Autoimmune hepatitis A form of liver inflammation.

Autonomic nerves Refers to peripheral nerves that carry signals from the brain and control such involuntary actions in the body as the beating of the heart.

Autonomic neuropathy affects the nerves that control heartbeat, blood pressure, sweating, digestion, urination, and sexual function.

Blood pressure The measurement of blood pressure in the arteries as the heart pumps blood and when

Bone marrow The inner core of bone that produces red and white blood cells.

Capillaries Tiny blood vessels that distribute oxygen-rich blood to the body and removes deoxygenated blood and waste. The smallest blood vessels in the circulatory system, they connect arteries to veins.

Carbohydrates Complex and simple (refined) sugars and starches that are broken down into glucose during digestion.

Cardiovascular disease Refers to diseases of the heart, arteries, capillaries, and veins.

Cardiovascular system The system of organs that include the the heart, arteries, capillaries, and veins. Also called the Circulatory System.

Cataracts is the clouding of the lenses of the eyes.

Cell The cell is the structural and functional unit of all known living organisms. It is the smallest unit of an organism that is classified as living, and is sometimes called the building block of life.

Cholesterol A chemical called a lipid that the body uses to make cell membranes and some hormones. HDL cholesterol (high density lipoprotein), is generally referred to as good cholesterol; LDL cholesterol (low density lipoprotein), is generally referred to as bad cholesterol.

Cirrhosis Scarring and damage of the liver cells and interruption of blood flow through the liver that leads to liver failure.

Coronary artery disease A condition in which sticky deposits (plaques) block the flow of blood to the heart, often causing chest pain (angina).

Cordiosteroid Powerful steroid used as an anti-inflammatory medication that reduces inflammation. It is also a steroid produced by the adrenal glands.

Cushing's syndrome is a condition that produces complications such as osteoporosis, high blood pressure, and roundness of the face. It is a condition characterized by an overproduction of adrenal gland secretions.

Diabetes is short for the disease called diabetes mellitus, a chronic disease associated with abnormally high levels of sugar in the blood. A disease in which the body cannot produce insulin or cannot use insulin to its full potential.

Diabetic nephropathy Damage to the kidney and impairment of kidney function which can lead to chronic renal failure, and can eventually require dialysis.

Dialysis An artificial way of cleansing the body by removing waste products from the blood and excess fluid from the body when the kidneys have failed.

Fasting blood sugar level Excessive output of glucose from the liver contributes to a high fasting blood sugar level.***

Fibromyalgia is chronic stiffness and paint in muscles, joints and tendons.

Fibrosis A formation or buildup of scar tissue on the liver.

Gangrene The death and decay of body tissue, most often caused by a loss of blood flow, especially in the legs, feet, and toes.

Gastroparesis Slow digestion and delayed emptying of the stomach due to nerve and muscle damage.

Glucagon A hormone produced by the pancreas that raises blood glucose levels.

Glucose a form of sugar in the bloodstream that is the body's primary fuel; glucose broken down from food can be converted into energy.

Glycogen is the converted form of glucose that is stored in the liver and muscles of the body. The liver converts it back to glucose to be used as energy.

Glycogenolysis is the metabolic process in which glycogen is broken down into glucose molecules.

Glycogenesis is the process by which glycogen is formed from glucose.

Granulomas are small lumps that form in tissues as the result of a collection of inflammatory cells. The cells collect because of an abnormal immune system response.

HDL Cholesterol also called good cholesterol removes deposits from the inner lining of blood vessels.

Heart. The heart is a muscular organ responsible for pumping blood through the blood vessels by repeated, rhythmic contractions.

Heart disease Any of a number of diseases related to the heart and blood vessels. Also known as coronary artery disease.

Hepatic Relating to or affecting the liver

Hyperglycemia is a condition in which the blood glucose level is higher than normal.

Hypertension The medical term for high blood pressure, where the blood circulates through the arteries with too much force.

Hypoglycemia is an abnormally low glucose level in the blood which is often due to too much insulin or too little glucose.

Immune system is the defense mechanism of the body that defend against infection, disease, and foreign substances.

Immunosuppressant A medication that suppresses the body's natural immune response.

Insulin A hormone secreted by the pancreas to control the amount of sugar in the blood.

Intestines are two digestive organs in the abdomen; the small intestines remove nutrients from the food to be used for energy, and the large intestines absorb water from the digested food, and make stool.

Ketoacidosis is the presence of high levels of ketones in the body, a result of uncontrolled diabetes.

Kidneys The two bean-shaped organs located below the ribs toward the middle of the back that filter wastes from the blood and form urine.

Lactic Acidosis is the presence of high levels of lactic acid in the body along with a low pH balance of the bloodstream.

LDL Cholesterol high levels of LDL Cholesterol increases the risk of heart disease as it builds up on the inner walls of blood vessels, narrowing the arteries.

Liver The liver is a large organ in the body that stores and metabolizes nutrients, destroys toxins and produces bile.

Liver failure Liver failure is the inability of the liver to perform its normal function.

Lungs. The lungs are a pair of breathing organs located with the chest which remove carbon dioxide from and bring oxygen to the blood

Lupus, also known as Systemic Lupus Erythematosus (SLE); an autoimmune disease that can affect any organ or system in the body.

Lymph Fluid composed of lymphocytes that provides cells with oxygen, food, and water.

Lymph nodes Small oval gland that makes up part of the immune system that removes germs, bacteria and, foreign particles from the body.

Lymphatic system A network of vessels carrying lymph to and from lymph nodes, the spleen, and thymus. Part of the immune system.

Malar rash is a red, blotchy facial rash, also called a butterfly rash that forms on the cheeks and across the bridge of the nose.

Metabolism A process where substances are broken and synthesized to convert food into energy.

Methotrexate An anti-inflammatory drug which suppresses the immune system.

Nephrons Parts of the kidney that filter the blood and remove waste products from the blood.

Nervous system The system of nerves, the spinal cord, and brain. It regulates and coordinates all the body's activities.

Neuropathy An abnormal and usually degenerative state of the peripheral nerves that results in pain, numbness, tingling, swelling, and muscle weakness in various parts of the body.

Nonalcoholic steatohepatitis (NASH) Inflammation of the liver and accumulation of fat in the liver cells.

Obesity The condition of being extremely overweight, or an accumulation of body fat.

Ostoearthritis is the breakdown and loss of cartilage in the joints, usually affects people after middle age.

Pancreas is an organ that produces the insulin hormone needed to regulate blood sugar levels, and produces enzymes to aid in the digestion of proteins, carbohydrates and fats.

Peripheral nerves Nerves that run from your brain and spinal cord to all other parts of your body.

Peripheral neuropathy is damage to peripheral nerves, the nerves that sense pain, hot, cold, and touch. These muscles also control muscle movement and strength. The peripheral nerves in the lower legs and feet are most commonly affected by diabetes.

Platelets are cells found in the blood that are needed to control bleeding and clotting.

Plaque A fatty buildup of substances on the inside walls of a blood vessel.

Plaquenil anti-inflammatory drug used in the treatment of rheumatoid arthritis and lupus.

Prednisone A corticosteroid, a powerful anti-inflammatory drug.

Red blood cells Blood cells that carry oxygen to tissues throughout the body.

Renal failure The loss of the kidneys function of filtering the blood, usually due to diabetes or other diseases.

Rheumatoid arthritis an autoimmune condition where the immune system attacks the joints, causing swelling and damage to the joints and can lead to disability.

Sarcoidosis is an inflammatory disease that can affect almost any organ in the body. It causes heightened immunity which means that a person's immune system, which normally protects the body from infection and disease, overreacts, resulting in damage to the body's own tissues.

Sleep apnea is a temporary suspension of breathing occurring repeatedly during sleep that often affects overweight people or those having an obstruction in the breathing tract. Symptoms include loud snoring, snorting and choking sounds at night.

Steatosis is another name for fatty liver (a build up of fat in the liver).

Synovial membrane is a layer of connective tissue that lines the joints. The synovial membrane creates a lubricating substance called synovial fluid.

Triglyceride A type of fat that consists of one glycerol and three fatty acids that is normally present in the blood. High levels of triglycerides are linked to heart disease and atherosclerosis.

Veins are blood vessels that carry blood from throughout the body back to the heart.

White blood cells The blood cells responsible for fighting infection. Also called leukocytes

Bibliography /
Recommended Reading

Alterman, Seymour L. *How to Control Diabetes.* Hollywood, FL. Lifetime Books, 1996.

American Diabetes Assosiation. American Diabetes Association Complete Guide to Diabetes. Alexandria, VA, A Bantam Book/published by arrangement with the American Diabetes Association, 1999.

American Diabetes Association and National Institute of Diabetes, Digestive, and Kidney Disease. The prevention or delay of type 2 diabetes. *Diabetes Care.* 2002:25(4):742-49.

Atlas, Nava. *Vegan Express.* New York, Broadway Books, 2008.

Beaser, Richard S., M.D., and Campbell, Amy P., R.D., M.S., CDE. The *Joslin Guide to Diabetes.* New York, Simon & Schuster, 2005.

Good Living With Osteoarthritis. Atlanta, Georgia, The Arthritis Foundation, 2006.

Barnard, Neal. *Diabetes Care,* August 2006; vol 29: pp 177-1783. News release, Physicians DCommittee for Responsible Medicine.

Barnard, Neal and Grogan, Bryanna Clark. *Dr. Neal Barnard's Program for Reversing Diabetes: The Scientifically Proven System for Reversing Diabetes Without Drugs.* New York, Rodale Books, 2007.

Becker, Gretchen, and Goldfine, Allison B. *The First Year: Type 2 Diabetes: An Essential Guide for the Newly Diagnosed.* New York, Marlow and Company, 2001.

Bernatsky, Sasha, M.D. and Senecagl, Jean-Luc, M.D., FRCPC, FACR. *Lupus, Everything You Need To Know.* New York, Firefly Books, 2005.

Bernstein, Richard K. Dr. Bernstein's Diabetes Solution: The Complete Guide to Achieving Normal Blood Sugars. New York, Little, Brown, and Company, 2007.

Bierman, June, and Toohey, Barbara. *The Diabetics Book.* New York, Penguin Putnam, Inc., 1998.

Bird, Howard, Green, Caroline, Hamer, Andrew, Hammond, Alison, Harkness, Janet, Hurley, Mike, Jefferson, Paula, Pattison, Dorothy, and Scott, David L. *Arthritis, Your Questions Answered.* New York, DK Publishing, 2007.

Blereav, Jude. *Whole Food, Heal, Nourish, Delight.* Australia, Murdoch Books, 2006.

Bortz, Walter M. II, M.D. *DiabetesDanger.* New York, Select Books, 2005.

Broadhurst, C. Leigh, PhD. *Diabetes Prevention and Cure.* New York, Kensington Books, 1999.

Budwig, Johanna. *Flax Oil as a True Aid Against Arthritis, Heart Infarction, Cancer, and Other Diseases.* Apple Publishing, Vancouver BC, 1994.

Centers for Disease Control. National Diabetes Fact Sheet *http://www.cdc.gov/diabetes/pubs/estimates.htm*, 2003

Chan, J.M., E B. Rimm, G.A. Colditz, M.J. Stampfer, and W.C Willett. Obesity, fat distribution, and weight gain as risk factors for clinical diabetes in men. *Diabetes Care*. 1994;17(9):961-9.

Chandalia, M., A. Garg, D. Lutjohann, K. Von Bergmann, S.M. Grundy, and L.J. Brinkley. Beneficial effects of high dietary fiber intake in patients with type 2 diabetes melliutus. New England Journal of Medicine. 2000;342:1392-98.

Cherewatenko, Vern, M.D., and Perry, Paul. *The Diabetes Cure*. New York, Harper Collins, 2000.

Clough, John D., M.D. *The Cleveland Clinic Guide to Arthritis*. NewYork, Kaplan Publishing, 2009.

Convit, A., O.T. Wolf, C. Tarshish, and M. J. de Leon. Reduced glucose tolerance is associated with poor memory performance and hippocampal atrophy among normal elderly. Proceedings of the National Academy of Sciences. 2003.

David, Brenda, RD. and Meliina, Vesanto, MS, RD. *Becoming Vegan*. Summertown, TN, Book Publishing, 2000.

Diabetes: Can a Vegan Diet Reverse Diabetes? Nicholson, Andrew, M. D. February 15, 2005. August 27, 2008. <http://www.pcrm.org/health/clinres/diabetes.html>;

The Diabetes Prevention Program (DPP) Research group. Reduction in the incidence of type 2 diabetes with lifestyle intervention or metformin. New England Journal of Medicine. 2002;346:393-403.

Diamond, Harvey, and Diamond, Marilyn. *Fit For Life*. New York, Grand Central Publishing, 1987.

Erasmus, Udo. Fats That Heal, Fats That Kill. Alive Books, Burnaby BC, 1993.

Erdmann, Robert, PhD. <u>Fats That Can Save Your Life.</u> Progressive Health Publishing, Encinitas, CA, 1995.

Fletcher, Ben, Penman, Danny, and Pine, Karen. *The No Diet Diet, Do Something Different.* London, England, Orion Publishing Group, Ltd., 2007.

Fontanarosa, Phil B., MD, MBA< DeAngelis, Catherine D., MD, MPH, Wong, John E. L., MBBS, FACP. JAMA<u>, National University Health System, Singapore, Host Diabetes, Obesity Meeting.</u> *JAMA The Journal of the American Medical Association.* October 15, 2008. 1750-1751.

Food and Nutrition Board, Institute of Medicine. *Dietary Reference Intakes for Energy, Carbohydrate, Fiber, Fat, Fatty Acids, Cholesterol, Protein, and Amino Acids.* Washington, DC: National Academy Press, 2002.

Foster-Powell, K., S. H. A. Holt, and J. C. Brand-Miller. International table of glycemic index and glycemic load values: *American Journal of Clinical Nutrition.* 2002;76:5-56.

Harrington, Jill. *The Lupus Recovery Diet.* Mill Valley, CA, Harbor Point Publishing, 2007.

Hobbs, Suzanne Havala. *Get the Trans Fat Out.* New York, Three Rivers Press, 2006.

House, Franklin M.D., Seal, Stuart A., M.D., and Newman, Ian Blake. *The 30-Day Diabetes Miracle: Lifestyle Center of America's Complete Program to Stop Diabetes, Restore Health, and Build Natural Vitality.* New York, the Penguin Group, 2008.

Hu, F.B., R.M. van Dam, and S. Liu. Diet and risk of type 2 diabetes: the role of types of fat and carbohydrate, *Diabetologia.* 2001;44:805-17.

Ivy, J.L. role of exercise training in the prevention and treatment of insulin resistance and noninsulin dependent diabetes mellitus. *Sports Medicine.* 1997;24(5):321-26.

The Journal of the American Medical Association, <u>Acrylamide Intake and Breast Cancer Risk in Swedish Women.</u> Vol. 293 No. 11, March 16, 2005.

Kelly, Pat. *Coping with Diabetes.* New York, The Rosen Publishing Group, 1998.

Klein, Donna, *The Mediterranean Vegan Kitchen.* New York, Berkley Publishing Group, 2001.

Kowalski, Robert E. *The Blood Pressure Cure.* New Jersey, John Wiley & Sons, 2007.

Lappe, F.M. *Diet for a Small Planet, 10ᵗʰ Anniversary Edition.* New York: Ballantine Books, 1982.

Laliberte, Richard, <u>Stopping Diabetes In Its Tracks</u>, Pleasantville, New York/ Montreal: Readers Digest, 2002.

Leonard, C. H., AMA, MD. <u>The Concise Gray's Anatomy</u>, Wordworth Editions Ltd, Hertfordshire, 1997.

Liu, S., J.E. Manson, M.J. Stampfer, F.B. Hu, E. Giovannucci, G.A. Colditz, C.H. Hennekens, and W.C. Willet, A prospective study of whole-grain intake and risk of type 2 diabetes mellitus in US women, *American Journal of Public Health.* 200;90(9):1409-15.

Marcus, Erik. *Vegan, the New Ethics of Eating.* NY, McBooks Press, 1998.

McCann, Jennifer. *Vegan Lunchbox.* Philadelphia, PA, Da Capo Press Books, 2008.

McClure, Ed and Lisa. *Eat Your Way to a Healthy Life.* Florida, Siloam, A Strang Company, 2006.

Milchovich, Sue K., RN, BXN, CDE, and Dunn-Long, Barbara, *Diabetes Melitus.* Boulder, CO. Bull Publishing, 2007.

Montenon, J., P. Knekt, R. Jarvinene, A. Aromaa, and Reunanen Antti. Whole grain and fiber intake and the incidence of type 2 diabetes. *American Journal of Clinical Nutrition.* 2003:77(3):622-29.

Murray, Micharl, N.D., and Lyon, Michael, M.D. *Beat Diabetes Naturally.* USA, Rodale, 2006.

Nappier, Kristine, MPH, R.D., L.D. *Eat Away Diabetes.* New York, Prentice Hall Press, 2002.

National Institute of Diabetes and Digestive and Kidney Diseases. *Am I at Risk for Diabetes?* NIH publication No. 02-4805; May 2002 *http://www.niddk.nih.gov/health/diabetes/pubs/risk/risk.htm#7*

Neal D. Barnard, MD, Joshua Cohen, MD, David J.A. Jenkins, MD, PHD, Gabrielle Turner-McGrievy, MS, RD, Lise Gloede, RD, CDE, Brent Jaster, MD, Kim Seidkl, MS, RD, Amber A. Green, RD, and Stanley Talpers, MD. "A Low-Fat Vegan Diet Improved Glycemic Control and Cardiovascular Risk Factors in a Randomized Clinical Trial in Individuals With Type 2 Diabetes." Diabetes Care, Volume 29, Number 8, August 2006.

Nedley, Neil. *Proof Positive: How to Reliably Combat Disease and Achieve Optimal Health Through Nutrition and Lifestyle.* Nedley Publications.

Nolfi, Kristine, M.D. *Raw Food Treatment of Cancer.* Brushton, NY, TEACH Services, 1995.

Periera, M.A., D.R. Jacobs, J.J. Pins, S.K. Raatz, M.D. Gross, J.L. Slavin, and E.R. Seaquist. Effect of whole grains on insulin sensitivity in overweight hyperinsulinemic adults. *American Journal of Clinical Nutrition.* 2002.

Phillips, Robert H., M.D. *Coping With Osteo-Arthritis.* New York, Avery Publishing Group, 1989.

Pirello, Christina. *This Crazy Vegan Life*. New York, Penguin Group, 2008.

Quillin, Patrick, PhD, RD, CNS. *The Diabetes Improvement Program*. Leader Co., 2001.

Robbins, John. *Diet For A New America*. California, HJ Kramer and New World Library, 1987.

Siedell, J, C, Obesity, insulin resistance, and diabetes-a worldwide epidemic. *British Journal of Nutrition*, 2000;83:S5-S8.

Simopoulos, A.P. Essential fatty acids in health and chronic disease. *American Journal of Clinical Nutrition*. 1999;70:560S-69S.

Steward, H. Leighton, Bethea, Morrison C., M.D., Andrews, Sam S. Andrews, M.D., Balart, Luis A., M.D. *Sugar Busters, Cut Sugar to Trim Fat*. New York, Ballantine Publishing Group, 1998.

U.S. Department of Health and Human Services, Dietary Guidelines for Americans. http://www.health.gov/DietaryGuidelines. October 16, 2006.

Vad, Vijay, M.D. *Arthritis RX*. New York, Gotham Books, 2006.

Van Dam, R.M., E.B. Rimm, W.C. Willett, M.J. Stampfer, and F.B. Hu. Dietary patterns and risk for type 2 diabetes mellitus in U.S. men. *Annals of Internal Medicine*. 2002;136(3):201-09.

Vegan Diet May Treat Diabetes. CBS News. July 26, 2006. August 27, 2008. <http://www.cbsnews.com/stories/2006/07/26/health/webmd/printable1837927.shtml>;

The Vegetarian Society of the United Kingdom, Information Sheet. www.vegsoc.org/info/protein.html. January 10, 2009.

Wallace, Daniel J., M.D. *The Lupus Book.* New York, Oxford University Press, 2005.

Whitaker, Julian, M.D., <u>Reversing Diabetes</u>. New York: Warner Books, 2001.

Woodruff, S., and Saudek, C. The Complete Diabetes Prevention Plan. New York, NY: Penguin Group (USA) Inc. 2004.

Index

Edwards Brothers, Inc.
Thorofare, NJ USA
May 19, 2011